Pregnant Feelings:
Developing Trust in Birth

PREGNANT FEELINGS:
Developing Trust in Birth

Rahima Baldwin
Terra Palmarini Richardson

CELESTIAL ARTS
Berkeley, California

Celestial Arts
P.O. Box 7327
Berkeley, CA 94707

First Printing 1986

Cover and interior design by Ken Scott
Cover and interior photography by Harriette Hartigan
Typography by HMS Typography, Inc.

Made in the United States of America
Library of Congress No. 85-062305

ISBN: 0-89087-423-9

3   4   5   —   96   95   94

Preface to the Second Edition

Pregnant Feelings: Developing Trust in Birth has been revised to serve as an antidote to the skyrocketing cesarean rate (now nearly 25 percent and the fact that use of epidural anesthesia has reached its highest rate in ten years. The reason women, once again, are giving away birth is that they have no confidence in the process of birth or their body's ability to give birth.

We offer *Pregnant Feelings* as a tool to help women understand and release those attitudes and emotions about pregnancy and birth which keep them from birthing with the confidence and power that is rightfully theirs. The inner work and understanding suggested in this book can be an important part of a change of women's consciousness, and this will inevitably result in further changes in established birthing practices.

Women need to understand more than just the physiological process of birth (although if birth were conducted physiologically, there would be a great improvement as women would be encouraged to walk about during labor, eat and drink to keep up their strength, and squat to open the pelvis and bring the baby down). Women also need to understand how labor *feels,* how their own energy and the energy of the contractions will be different at two centimeters of dilation than at nine. When they understand the mind-body connection, they will appreciate the importance of the environment and their attitude on maintaining the hormonal levels for an effective labor complete with endorphins, nature's own pain relievers. Learning how to work *with* the process of birth is one of the primary ways of preventing unnecessary cesareans.

This book is designed to help pregnant women increase their confidence by exploring their ideas and emotions about pregnancy and birth, releasing unresolved emotions from previous experiences, and developing trust in their bodies and their abilities to give birth in their own unique ways. It can be used alone, shared with a partner or friend, or used in childbirth preparation classes to stimulate discussion.

It has been written out of our deep respect for women and the process of birth. As servants of birth, we have come to know its power and its myriad faces as it manifests in the family of women. Through our experiences as midwives, mothers, and childbirth educators, we have also seen how birth can be made more difficult through a woman's own fears and the medical system's view of birth as a dangerous disease from which women need to be delivered. Interventions that could have been avoided are costly both emotionally as well as physiologically. It is our hope that this book will contribute to women reclaiming birth as a process for which their bodies and minds are uniquely suited.

In writing *Pregnant Feelings: Developing Trust in Birth* we have drawn from more than two decades of combined experience in working with pregnant women, first as childbirth educators and then as midwives. Rahima became a childbirth educator in 1974, founded Informed Homebirth/Informed Birth and Parenting as a national educational organization, and wrote *Special Delivery* (Celestial Arts, 1979). She is a practicing midwife and co-director of the Garden of Life birth center in Dearborn, Michigan. She also has a counseling practice for dealing with birth-related experiences. She lives in Ann Arbor with her husband Agaf Dancy and three children.

Terra's work with women and personal growth began in college, where she studied psychology and participated in feminist consciousness-raising groups. With her own pregnancy, her interest in women's issues found expression in the field of birth. She became an Informed Homebirth instruction in 1980 and is a practicing midwife in Boulder, Colorado, where she began the ReSourcing Birth Midwifery School. She is co-president of the Colorado Midwives Association and a coauthor of the CMA Certification Program. She lives with her husband Charlie Richardson and two children.

Terra began writing *Pregnant Feelings* in 1979 when she was pregnant with her first child, Julien. Rahima, who had emphasized the psychological aspects of birth throughout her career, joined the project in 1984, and this book is the result of their combined efforts. It is a personal book so it is addressed to "you" and refers to "us" when both authors share a view or experience and to "Rahima" or "Terra" when talking about our individual experiences. We are glad to be sharing with you the adventure of pregnancy and birth and wish you an experience full of inner growth, vibrant health for you and your baby, and an increased sense of yourself as a woman.

Rahima Baldwin
Terra Palmarini Richardson
April, 1990

Table of Contents

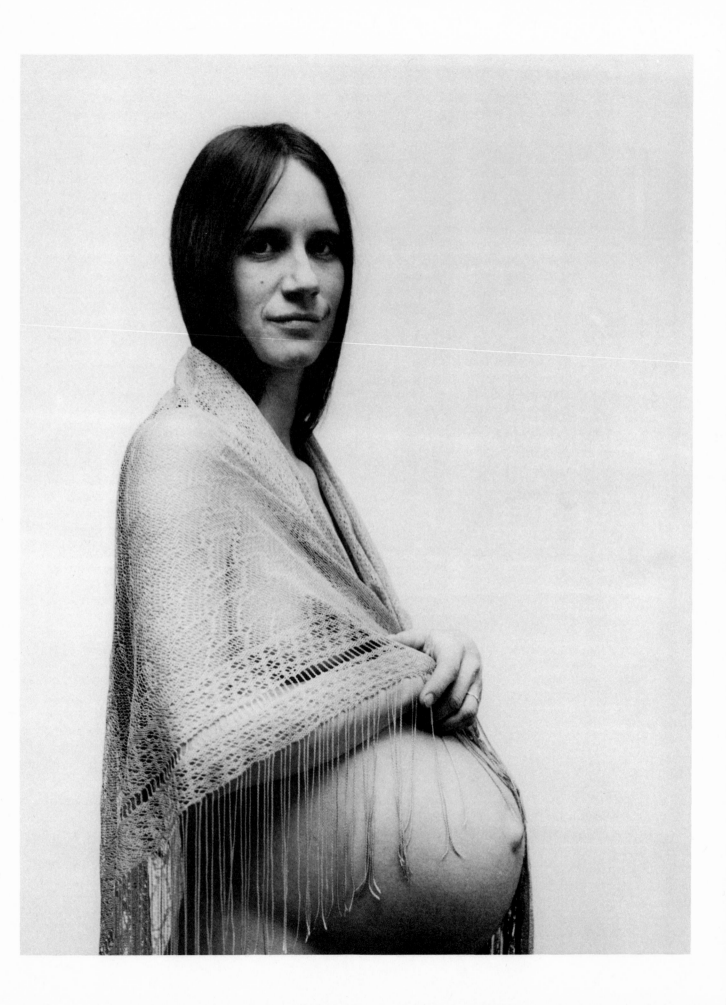

1
Trusting Birth

The Energy of Birth

For hundreds of years people have wondered what was behind Mona Lisa's enigmatic smile. In the photo at left we can see that Mona Lisa really was pregnant, looking out at us with all the wisdom and knowing which a pregnant woman embodies.

Most Western women today find it difficult to contact this deep inner knowing and trust in the process of birth. They are usually insulated from birth except for exaggerations in the media or unsettling stories from friends about their experiences in the hospital. The edpidural anesthesia rate in America is the highest it has been in ten years and the cesarean rate is almost 25 percent—that's "one in four if you walk in the door." Clearly something is missing as modern women once again absent themselves from one of the most powerful experiences of being a woman and turn birth over to the experts to do to them.

One of the things that keeps us from having confidence in our bodies and the process of birth is the sense that birth is bigger than we are. This is true—and can be frightening because forces are at work that are not under our control. When a woman opens herself to being pregnant, whether consciously or unconsciously, she becomes the vessel for new life, the pathway through which a new human being assumes physical form and joins life on this earth. Whether you feel that you are serving the preservation of the species, serving God, or serving the being of the child who is coming through you, your life stops being entirely your own. You must make way for another being, both within your body as your organs adjust to the growing baby, and within your awareness as you start to mother the child inside.

Being pregnant is getting on a train that whisks you down the track to a destination not precisely known. The changes that will occur in a woman's body, emotions, and relationships are unknown. So is the sex of the baby and his or her character and destiny, except as they are revealed in intuitions, dreams, or that latest necessity called ultrasounds.

Because pregnancy is a time of so many changes—both physical and emotional—it can be a time of tremendous inner growth. Emotions and one's own "inner child" are very close to the surface and they are ripe for growth. The exercises in this book that deal with emotions can help you experience the joys of pregnancy and birth, but they are not absolutely necessary. Your baby is going to be born regardless! You don't have to be psychologically clear to give birth without assistance from anesthesia, pitocin, forceps, or surgery.

All you have to do is open to the energy of birth and work with it. If you don't block it, it will birth your baby. You won't be given more than you can bear, although at the point of surrender in labor, you may wonder. But that surrender to the energy of birth makes everything change and brings your baby out to your arms.

The energy of birth exists both apart from us and in us, just as sexual energy does. Together they are the energy of creation and we share in both, but we cannot keep them in our control like tamed animals. Just as the energy of sexual arousal requires surrender if orgasm is to occur, so the energy of birth requires surrender if the baby is going to come out without intervention. There must be an opening— an allowing or letting go—in the face of something more powerful than ourselves. It is possible to open with ecstasy, concentration, bellowing, or controlled breathing, but you must let labor come and welcome its increasing intensity.

Your body knows how to birth. You have to trust it and the natural process. You can't *learn* how to give birth, just as you can't learn how to sneeze or to have an orgasm. There has to be a letting go, an allowing it to happen. For it is often possible to stifle a sneeze or to block orgasm, and it is all too often possible to be at odds with the energy of birth.

A respect for the energy of birth has always existed among women, who have known its beauty and power in their own bodies and have passed on the ancient wisdom of birthing from one generation to the next. Indeed, the French word for midwife, *sage-femme,* also means "wise woman." Those of us who work as midwives know and appreciate the energy of birth, because we have had to work with heart and hands to help women release blocks when the birth energy has become stuck. Not wishing to resort to anesthesia, chemicals or instruments has helped us learn how to work with birthing women. They, and birth itself, have been our teachers.

Midwives from varied backgrounds have talked about the energy at birth. Ina May Gaskin, midwife at a community in Tennessee, describes contractions as "rushes" of energy and speaks extensively of ways women and attendants can work with the energy during labor and delivery.[1] Elizabeth Davis, in her book *Heart and Hands: A Midwife's Guide,* discusses various turning points in labor that require the mother to shift gears and take on more energy.[2] Midwife Iris Wolfson expresses an understanding of the flow of energy at a birth when she says, "To me every birth has its own logic and rhythm . . . . I am not advocating that we do away with interventions, but I think we should pay more attention to going with the flow of a particular labor, to observing the quality of any complication that arises, the way it unfolds. Too often we cut off the flow and force it to fit our own notions of what *should* be happening."[3]

Many midwifes are able to tell dilation (how far the cervix is open) just by the quality of the energy in the room rather than needing to do an internal exam. Certainly they take cues from everything they perceive—the color of the mother's cheeks, the nature of her gaze, the hardness of her belly during contractions, and her emotions—but they also don't invalidate their direct perception of the energy present. Jesusita Aragon, a 74-year-old midwife who has been at more than 15,000 births, started to yawn repeatedly at one point in a labor that Rahima was privileged to attend with her. When Rahima naively asked if she was tired and needed assistance, she said, "No, I always yawn when they are in transition." Sure enough, a few contractions later the head began to be visible. The energy during transition has a characteristic "sticky" quality for which yawning was her response.

The energy present at a birth is very powerful. Whether you believe that it is generated by the increasingly strong contractions of the uterus or is the cause of them, the fact that a tremendous amount of energy flows through a woman giving birth is hard to deny. Sometimes a woman giving birth is hard to deny. Sometimes a woman can feel as if she has used the energy required for a 50-mile hike; other times she feels as if a tremendous force has swept through her and left her startled to be holding her baby after so short a time. Whether a labor is long or short, the creation of a new life is always stunning. Once, during a three-hour labor in the middle of the afternoon, Rahima thought, "This birth ought to be easy to recover from." But she and everyone present were as exhausted as if it had been a long labor in the middle of the night. Going through birth with a woman is always a profoundly involving event, touching very deep places within us.

Thinking about the energy of birth as something which is at once within and outside of the birthing woman eliminates debate over whether it is a manifestation of a biochemical process caused by the changing hormones in the woman's body or whether there is a creative life force in the universe that is greated than the individuals who participate in it. Philosophical explanations aren't as useful as simply recognizing the energy, honoring it, and learning how to work with it.

Western medicine has taken a very mechanical view of the human being, regarding the human body as a "wonderful machine" whose systems function together like a complex factory. When organs break down, the repairman can be called to fix or even replace them without regard for the "owner's" participation or responsibility for the system as a whole. In other cultures, systems of medicine that have not developed out of the dissection of corpses nor encompassed the possibility of easy surgery, have had to work with the human being's connection to the energy that surrounds and flows through the body, and with the interrelatedness of body, mind and spirit. These approaches are becoming accepted by Western medicine, so that some doctors are beginning to incorporate elements of Chinese, aurovedic or homeopathic medicine into their practices. In one stunning example, Dolores Krieger, professor of nursing at New York University, has trained more than 8000 health professionals in what has come to be called "Therapeutic Touch." This evolved out of her doctoral investigation of the "laying on of hands," which she explains in terms of the Sanskrit word *prana* (life force), which can be transferred through one person to another to aid in healing.[4]

Touch is one obvious way to facilitate the flow of energy during labor and delivery, since it releases tension and aids relaxation. Krieger's work has been taught in childbirth education classes and is especially suited to hospital birth because no physical touching is actually involved. It has resulted in increased relaxation of both the woman and her coach, increased awareness of the baby during pregnancy, and improvement of the couple's marital relationship.[5]

In addition to touch, other factors that can aid or impede the flow of energy during labor and delivery include the mother's preparation and ability to relax and open, her position, her relationship with her partner, the attitudes and sensitivity of the people attending her, and the physical environment. The importance of the environment is known and honored with animals, for it has been observed that if a mother animal is disturbed during labor, the labor will be longer and there will be more stillborn young; if she doesn't feel safe, labor will actually stop.[6] Dr. Michel Odent, whose work with birth is described in Chapter 4, has tried to create an environment in which a woman can contact her deeper, instinctual knowledge about birthing and give birth in her own way with a minimum of intervention. He has found that the conditions conducive to making love are also best for birthing and has created a birthing room with low lighting and a platform mattress that does not restrict the woman to any one position for birthing. He writes, "To sum up, privacy, intimacy, calm, freedom to labor in any position, and the helpful presence of midwives are crucial to a spontaneous first-stage of labor."[7]

But Odent is the exception among doctors, because unfortunately most don't even recognize that there is a change in the energy at a birth.[8] This is because they don't sit with a woman through all the variations of labor, but come for occasional visits and to do the "important work" at the end. When Rahima offered a workshop at a local hospital on working with the energy of birth, nurses, childbirth educators and labor-support people were eager to learn ways they could be more helpful to women in birth. No doctors attended, and one angrily told the sponsor, "What is all this (expletive deleted) about birthing energy? There's no such thing!" The immensity of the chasm that can exist between birthing women and the health care system is illustrated by statements such as those by Dr. Robert Sokol, professor and chairman of Ob-Gyn at Wayne State University and Hutzel Hospital in Detroit. He was quoted in the Detroit News as saying, "The vagina is not made for having babies any more than the penis is."[9] Not only are such attitudes absurd in the extreme, they have resulted in obstetrics becoming a specialized branch of surgery.

Even when doctors genuinely respect women and want to help them in birth, they are often blind to the energy involved. Dr. Michael Collins, head of obstetrics at Munson Hospital in Traverse City, Michigan said, "I see us working real hard to get women to deliver vaginally, and we're just amazed that they can't."[10] Only a lack of perception on the part of doctors and complacency on the part of women can sustain a way of birthing that violates the interaction of mind and body, not to mention the laws of gravity.

The predicament we find ourselves in today is that women feel isolated and cut off from their bodies, as well as from their connection with all other women who have given birth throughout time. The way of birthing in our country follows the male model of dominance and control, which women have agreed to out of fear and a desire to be taken care of. Through fear and ignorance, women of our mothers' generation allowed themselves to be knocked out completely while birth was performed on them by doctors. Today, general anesthesia is rarely used, due to risks for the mother and baby, but the continued management and manipulation of women in labor has led to their subordination to machines, timetables and technology. Awake and aware, they have nevertheless become spectators at their own children's births.

But change is in the air. Women are waking up to the fact that the current cesarean rate of nearly 25 percent nationally and 45 percent in some large teaching hospitals is more a result of the model of birth we practice than any inherent flaws in their own physiology. Even if they don't end up with a cesarean, women often feel as if they have been manhandled during what should have been a profound experience in their lives. The suspicion exists that there has to be a better way. That way involved women reclaiming their bodies and their births, becoming the active givers of birth, and taking responsibility for seeing that those who attend them work with them and respect their unique way of giving birth.

This book is designed to increase your familiarity with the energy of birth and those attitudes and actions that tend to encourage its flow. The exercises that deal with emotions are designed to help you let go of fears and past experiences that block the free flow of energy and to increase your confidence in your own inner wisdom and ability to birth.

As the book progresses you'll gain an understanding of how the energy tends to flow during labor and delivery, things you and your attendants can do to work with it, and ways of removing blocks should they arise. You'll also be able to explore your feelings about pregnancy and birth and let go of emotional blocks or holding which you may bring from past experiences.

Before turning to the emotional aspects of pregnancy, we'd like you to try an exercise in which you imagine that you could have a conversation with the energy of birth that we have been discussing. Personify this energy enough to imagine a dialogue between yourself and "Birthing Energy." In this way you can express any questions about birth that may have been concerning you, or you may find that there is a "message" for you. If you have a question, start with it—or just say "Hi!" and see where things go. You can do this exercise whether you are a man or a woman, pregnant or not. Take the next ten minutes for a "Dialogue with Birthing Energy."

Write what comes to you as a dialogue between yourself and a force that you call Birthing Energy. Refer to yourself as "Me" and to Birthing Energy as "B.E." It doesn't matter who starts first. It could be a greeting or a question, or maybe the energy wants to say something to you. Don't skip this exercise, but don't agonize over it—just write what comes to you. Less thinking and more writing.

Me: _____

_____

B.E.: _____

_____

Me: _____

_____

B.E.: _____

_____

Me: _____

_____

B.E.: _____

_____

What was your experience with this exercise? In thinking in this way about the energy of birth, did it seem masculine or feminine or simply like a force? This exercise was developed by Penny Camp, an Informed Homebirth teacher in Atlanta, and is designed to show you that you carry the answers to your own questions within you.

Throughout the book we will share dialogues with Birthing Energy given to us by workshop participants. Those dealing with practical questions about previous births or the upcoming one will be included in later chapters. Here we want to share a few of the many dealing with the nature of the energy itself. You will notice that many people responded in spiritual terms, an indication of the profound nature of their feelings.

Various Women's Dialogues with Birthing Energy (B.E.)

Me: *I'm awed by your power.*
B.E.: *I am the power of the universe—the eternal flow.*
Me: *I fear your moving through me. I fear I'm not strong enough.*
B.E.: *You are a worthy channel. Openness is asked of you, not strength.*
Me: *My fears, the ancient wives' tales, they are as logs across a river damming the flow. What must I do so that the current may move freely?*
B.E.: *I am the source of ebb and flow of the universe. Trust that you are a part of that majesty and that I, in you, am in perfect order.*
Me: *Yes, but . . .*
B.E.: *My daughter, as the flowers open their ripening centers to the sun, so shall your center soon be opened. There is nothing to do but feel yourself as a channel. The sun is drawing forth the sweetness from your womb.*

Me: *We will get a second chance to meet. This time I will be more conscious and work with you.*
B.E.: *I am a strong force. If we work together and don't fight each other, things will be fine.*
Me: *I will trust your power and do my part—relax, breathe deeply, stay calm and feel every moment of the experience.*

B.E.: *That's good. I know what to do. I will trust you also and together we will birth this new being.*

Me: *You're here?*
B.E.: *Yes, and ready to go to work.*
Me: *Where do you come from?*
B.E.: *I come from within you, the source of life.*
Me: *What do you do?*
B.E.: *I focus all your inner energies toward the birthing and giving of a new life from within your body.*
Me: *Why are you sometimes so dreaded and feared?*
B.E.: *I am an enormous bottleneck of overwhelming energy, and I need positive feelings to help guide me in my direction. Negative attitudes work against my positive goal and cause conflict within.*

B.E.: *I've been here since the beginning.*
Me: *Are you picked up by people not giving birth?*
B.E.: *Yes. Sometimes when you see a flower bloom or a new day dawn or an infinite number of other things you experience me—for I'm the energy of creation.*
Me: *Friendly.*
B.E.: *Yes, but I'm not always felt as friendly. Sometimes a woman or a man fear me, misunderstand me, judge me. Then I become fragmented and less effective.*
Me: *What can help this fragmentation?*
B.E.: *Acceptance, love, awareness of me now—for I may change from moment to moment. I am there in doses you can deal with, one moment at a time. Refocus on my purpose: the birth, the passage of life. For I am a blessing and a gift.*

B.E.: *I am here, awaken.*
Me: *I'm breathing. I'm alive.*
B.E.: *Breathe, always breathe.*
Me: *So much more, so much more than I knew, than I anticipated . . .*
B.E.: *Expect nothing. Allow everything. I am life.*
Me: *I am alive. I am breathing. Just breathing and moaning.*

B.E.: *Deep sounds that echo me. My eternity. I am you. I am your life. I am life. I am your mother. I am cosmic fire. I am mother of all worlds. Hear me. Sound me. Let me be free and flowing. I live in light and in sound. I vibrate and pulse and establish the rhythms of all universes. Have no fear to echo my sounds, my rhythms, and my power.*

Me: *I'm crying with no reason, or all reasons, only pure emotion. Energy in motion. Moving me. Opening me. Freeing me. I am free. I am free. I am free.*

B.E.: *Breathe deeply. Center yourself. Don't get lost. The energy is here and now. Don't go anywhere. Stay here. I am here with you. I AM.*

Me: *I really don't know what to say to you.*
B.E.: *Why's that?*
Me: *Well, I guess I'm not sure who you are.*
B.E.: *Oh? Why's that?*
Me: *Well, I guess it's the way people talk about you.*
B.E.: *In what way?*
Me: *People talk like you're an entity in yourself. I guess I never thought of you as energy.*
B.E.: *Who do you think of me as?*
Me: *I guess I've known all along that you are not energy or a force, but a person; that you're involved in all aspects of my life and not just birth.*
B.E.: *Who am I then?*
Me: *The Holy Spirit whom Jesus promised and the prophets alluded to.*
B.E.: *So why are you still writing down "BE" before you quote me?*
Me: *Sorry, Lord. I guess it's just the confusion that comes from other people's misunderstanding of who you are and what you do. It obscured you to me for a minute there.*

Me: *What are you?*
B.E.: *I am the spirit of life. I am all beginnings.*
Me: *Where do you come from?*
B.E.: *I am from within you and I am from without. Without me all life would change. Not necessarily cease, but change. Birth, as you know it, would*

come *from other sources. I have been since the beginning of time and so I will be until the end. I am the force that moves all life. The desire to continue. Sometimes I am gentle; sometimes I am firm. I am gentle in the birth of an idea or a way of life. The energy is the same, only the way I manifest myself varies. In childbirth I am firm in that it is important to continue. It takes strength, physical strength to live in the flesh, so it must take strength to birth in the flesh. The flesh is weak, is too willing to give up, and I am what makes the flesh continue. I am the spirit and the desire of life.*

Me: *So you're what gets the baby out?*
B.E.: *Yup, what were you expecting, a forklift maybe?*
Me: *No, I guess not.*
B.E.: *So what did you think I'd look like?*
Me: *Oh, a big yellow-orange ball of light.*
B.E.: *Pretty good.*
Me: *Well, sometimes you're a dark cloud, too.*
B.E.: *It all depends on what you make of me.*
Me: *Why do some folks have such a hard time with you?*
B.E.: *Because they won't admit I'm just one more part of them.*
Me: *You mean you're really just a part of me?*
B.E.: *Of course!*

For a while we wondered if including these might offend those of you who aren't "religious." But there's no one who isn't spiritual, especially when pregnant. Pregnancy is a time of being in touch with the power of creation itself. We would like to encourage you at this special time in your life to stay in touch with your spirituality, whether that means individual prayer or meditation, or affiliating with a church, synagogue or other spiritual center.

We would also encourage you to do this exercise at various times throughout your pregnancy, for your questions will change, and so will the answers. This exercise can remind you that you hold the answers within, that you have access to your own intuitive nature in your relationship with birth. We will include other women's words in response to this exercise at various places throughout this book.

Growth and Emotions in Pregnancy

Pregnancy is a time of growth. The growth of the baby is obvious, as is the changing profile of the mother. But the psychological development of the mother, and secondarily of the father, during this time make pregnancy a period of evolution unparalleled in a person's life. Body, roles, sexual drive, fears, appetites, sleep patterns and more are shifting. Some changes can be predicted with certainty, while others are only likely—or even surprising—making each pregnancy a unique event.

Changes can be exciting, like the first time the baby's movements are felt, or alarming, as in the unfamiliar cramping of the uterus. They are always easier to handle with the help of knowledge and relaxation, but pregnancy and giving birth rank near the top of the list as causes of stress in a person's life. The amount of stress is directly proportional to how well we handle and adapt to new situations.

The transitional time of pregnancy is one of preparation for the new state of motherhood that will inexorably arrive. Increased maturity is called for, even demanded. Fortunately nature has provided us with the possibility of increased emotional growth during this time. A pregnant woman's connection with the energy of creation and the hormonal changes in her body make her emotions much closer to the surface, much more accessible, more fluid and more strongly felt. It is easier for a woman to be in touch with her own "inner child" during this time, and therapists speak enthusiastically about the rapid growth and insights of women when they are pregnant.

The same is true for the expectant father, but to a lesser degree, since he lacks the sense of immediacy that a growing baby brings to a woman's body and emotions. But the changes in his partner, the presence of the baby as it becomes real to him, the reminders of his own parents, and his feelings about increased responsibility and fathering all make emotional growth more possible than at times of relative ease.

The third person whom the emotions of pregnancy involve is the child. The emotional state of the mother is translated into her physical body, the home environment of the baby. The baby is affected not only in utero, as the work of Verny and others has shown, but also through the impact of emotions on the birth experience.[11] For example, a mother who unconsciously feels that she "deserves" a cesarean because of a past abortion will create a very different experience for the baby than a woman who feels she deserves a supportive attendant and a fully natural birth experience.

In addition, the way parents feel about the birth influences their actions in parenting and how they feel about themselves as parents. Work at counselling centers and our own experiences have confirmed that how a woman feels about her birth influences how she feels about her parenting experience. Conversely, clearing emotions about a past birth experience can result in inceased closeness and a clearer relationship with the child in the present.

The time of pregnancy can be used by mothers and fathers to develop parenting values and skills. This time allows parents to accept their child as part of themselves and also to begin letting go of it (allowing it to be born separate from them), the two basic movements of the Dance of Parenthood.

In some cultures, older children are initiated into child care by learning to care for younger siblings and relatives. Many of us, however, have to take on the job of parenting self-consciously as adults with little or no practice experience. In this case, the nine months of gestation offer a chance to evaluate ourselves, to decide what we need to know more about, and to follow through in those areas.

All of the disruptions and inconveniences of pregnancy can be seen as natural psychological preparation for parenthood. Looking on them in this way may help turn them into lessons rather than tribulations. Responsibility and discipline may be cultivated in following exercise, nutrition or relaxation regimens. Patience may be developed in waiting for the birth to begin and then for labor to be over. For example, toward the end of Terra's pregnancy, she felt as if she were being turned into a baby herself—eating many small meals, getting colic, waking in the night to go to the bathroom and to get a drink. It helped her a great deal to view it as a way of better understanding her coming baby.

It is possible consciously to take advantage of this time of heightened emotional growth. Inner work can be done alone, shared with a friend, or done together as a couple. *Pregnant Feelings* is designed for all three modes of exploration. We suggest that you do the exercises individually; write your own responses and then share them with your partner or a friend. Assuming you are in a marriage or primary relationship, we suggest that you then ask your partner to do the exercises that are specifically for men.

Then discuss your answers and reactions. In this way you will grow as a couple as well as individually. Pregnancy brings on a wealth of opportunities to become more aware of ourselves, and thus to use all of our energies to the utmost—a must when parenting.

The Power of Emotions

The power of the emotions surrounding pregnancy and birth cannot be underestimated. During labor they are felt with such urgency and intensity that they usually stay with a woman the rest of her life. Talking with an older woman about her birthing experience often evokes a description charged with all the emotions of forty years earlier. Giving birth is a major event in a woman's life. It can be fulfilling and lead to enhanced self-esteem, or it can leave bitterness or unresolved emotions that last a lifetime. The more than 40,000 letters that Nancy Wainer Cohen, founder of C/SEC, received from cesarean mothers all over the country bear witness to the fact that women cannot be treated as objects without objecting.[12] Our feelings about ourselves and our births affect how we look, feel and relate to our partners and children.

Releasing past emotions and resolving fears about the upcoming birth can result in a more positive, fulfilling experience of pregnancy, with increased vitality and well-being for both mother and child. Emotional events trigger reactions within the mother's body that are chemically transmitted to the fetus. The hormones of the fight-or-flight reaction or the hormones of relaxation reach the baby during its development. These hormones also affect the unborn baby by influencing its environment in the womb. Relaxation allows for the best flow of blood and the best all-around environment for a healthy, growing baby.

The emotional state of a woman during pregnancy can also affect the kind of choices she makes about birth attendants and where to give birth. Someone who always feels powerless around authority figures is more likely to choose a doctor who says he'll take care of everything than is a woman who knows that she is responsible for herself and actively works with her doctor or midwife to create the kind of experience she wants.

The premise of this book—that it *is* possible to affect what happens to you, physically as well as emotionally—is well-supported by the work of Simonton and others in helping "terminally ill" cancer patients recover,[13] and by the work of Peterson and Mehl, who have predicted complications of labor with 95 percent accuracy based on a woman's total health profile, emotional and physical.[14] While we cannot predict with absolute certainty what will happen to us or how labor will go, it is possible to influence our experiences without blaming ourselves if we have a complication (or if a nurse looks cross-eyed at us!). There can be responsibility without blame. This is an attitude that enables us to be co-creators in life as it unfolds, attracting the most positive and life-giving events to ourselves. Other times we see that we have cooperated in things we don't like but then realize that what we learned from such experiences has profoundly affected our inner growth.

A mother's emotional state can affect the speed and ease of her work during labor. Grantly Dick-Read, in his pioneering classic on natural childbirth, *Childbirth Without Fear* explained the "Fear-Tension-Pain Triangle."[15] Fear during childbirth can cause tension and inhibition of the blood flow to the uterus, as well as involuntary constriction of the circular muscle layer of the uterus. This tightening resists the opening action of the longitudinal muscles, and working against oneself in this way can lead to true pain and an escalating cycle of fear, tension and pain. For this reason Dick-Read emphasized the supreme importance of prenatal education and relaxation for childbirth.

More recently, Gayle Peterson explained in her book, *Birthing Normally,* how repressed anger and fears, as well as certain reactive attitudes in pregnant women, are related to physical problems in labor such as prolonged labor or hemorrhage.[16] Her work in holistic prenatal care shows that awareness and counselling during pregnancy can help improve many women's self-image and birth outcome.

Emotions influence our body, our health, our weight, our body armor, and the way in which we make love and give birth. There is no right way to give birth, just as there is no right way to make love. There is no question of failure, although it is amazing how often women feel like failures when they could be feeling ecstatic about having given birth. Working with emotions is not going to guarantee you a short, easy labor. In fact, we have known women who were very upset after short labors because they felt they didn't behave properly during the surprising intensity of the contractions; and women with very long labors have been satisfied, feeling that they finally accomplished something at which they worked extremely hard. Work with emotions can help you to understand yourself so that growth can continue. But it can't offer any guarantees.

With all the emphasis on pregnancy and birth, it is necessary to remind ourselves that pregnancy has a finite limit. Birth itself, although tremendously powerful and important from the standpoint of the one who is pregnant, is but a doorway to parenthood, which has the everydayness and lack of glamour requiring all the stamina and skills one can muster. Having a new baby results in a tremendous transformation of lifestyle created by interrupted sleeping patterns, 24-hour responsibility, and so forth. Inner struggle is often required to maintain equanimity in the face of a colicky baby who will not allow herself to be put down.

The impact of emotions on parenting is clearly seen with breastfeeding, where feelings of fear, embarrassment, worry and anxiety can inhibit the let-down reflex and thus seriously restrict the amount of milk which the baby gets. This is more likely to occur at the beginning of breastfeeding a new baby, before the reflex has been firmly conditioned to respond to the infant's sucking and before the new mother has established confidence in the process of breastfeeding. Relaxation is especially important to breastfeeding for this reason.

As a pregnant woman, you are involved in an intimate relationship with the energy of creation. It will grow and birth your baby, and give birth to you as a new mother. The beauty and intensity of life is manifesting through you during your pregnancy, and even more strongly during the hours of labor to come. In the face of this, emotions are generated that can help or hinder the work of birth. We want to help you identify what you are feeling now, understand how the past impinges upon the present, and explore ways of clearing up traumas so they aren't likely to repeat. Then you can look forward to creating a birth experience that is emotionally fulfilling and results in "a healthy baby and a healthy mother." The tools and skills thus developed can then be turned toward the postpartum period and parenting. Let's begin!

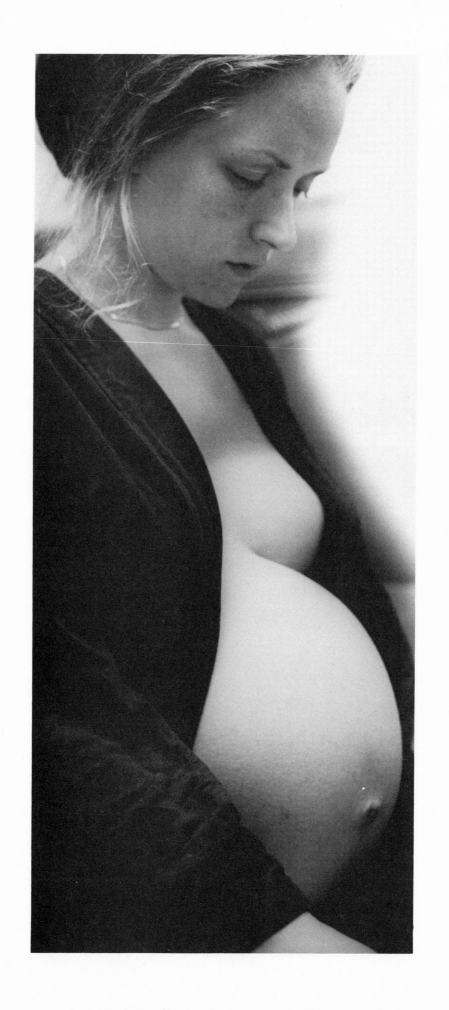

2
Changing Feelings /
Feeling Changes

Knowing Your Feelings

This chapter begins to explore how you feel about your baby, your body, your sexuality, your partner—and about giving birth. First let's look at the whole realm of emotions, naming feelings and making an emotional profile. The beginning exercises may seem very simple, but important insights can be hidden in them.

Naming Feelings

Feelings are a powerful force in our lives, whether or not we recognize them. But, to use their energy consciously in beneficial ways, we must learn to recognize what they are. Unnamed anger may come out as angry actions, such as kicking the dog or yelling at the children, and then blaming them for making us do it. Unnamed frustration may build up tension in the shoulders, as though you are carrying the weight of the world. Feeling hurt or threatened can manifest itself as anger and belligerence unless the real emotions are acknowledged. Unnamed fears can lead to superstitious behaviors or grasping onto an authority figure to take the responsibility for what happens.

Recognizing feelings can come from just being aware of how we feel, or it can come through evaluating what motivates us. Why exactly did we kick the dog? What or whom would we rather have kicked, and why?

Practice noticing your emotions by observing how your body reacts in various situations. What does your breathing do? What does your heart do? Are you flushed? Are your hands tense? Your jaw? Your shoulders? Learn to recognize your own physical signals of emotions.

Name three emotional situations where you have practiced noticing your physical reactions, and list at least three reactions for each situation.

Situation

I was feeling: _____

_____

_____

_____

My body reacted by: _____

_____

_____

_____

Situation

I was feeling: _____

_____

_____

_____

My body reacted by: _____

_____

_____

_____

Situation

I was feeling: _____

_____

_____

_____

My body reacted by: _____

_____

_____

_____

As you go through the following list of emotions, try to act, look and feel each one. Recall situations in which you felt the emotion, or simply imagine a situation in which you would feel it. In what situation(s) might you have each feeling? Is it a familiar feeling? Do you enjoy it?

cheerful	unhappy	proud	crowded
joyful	guilty	fearless	jealous
forgiving	fretful	sad	despairing
used	judgmental	repelled	tired
irritated	humble	empty	alone
delighted	fearful	vain	unsuccessful
thankful	beautiful	ridiculous	modest
authoritative	spiritual	sexy	ugly
happy	hostile	glamorous	triumphant
annoyed	angry	sociable	confident
centered	relieved	alienated	friendly
arrogant	passive	plain	optimistic
grateful	generous	active	peaceful

Which ones in the list did you want to avoid trying on? Circle the five most familiar and underline the five least familiar.

Pregnancy, with its heightened emotions, often brings us in touch with feelings that don't fit our self-image, our accepted range of feelings. An inner attitude of acceptance can help such feelings pass quickly or help parts of ourselves grow and transform. During pregnancy you might feel anger or dependency that you haven't felt since you were a little girl. When you accept these feelings rather than being afraid of them you allow inner breathing and growth. Thus, remembering can be "re-membering," a bringing together of parts of ourselves that have been locked away in dark rooms.

Profiles of Pregnancy

The following exercise is to be done separately by you and your partner. Take ten minutes or less to write the answers to the following questions. Write quickly, answering with whatever comes to you rather than pondering whether that's what you really feel. This is a "whatever comes into your head" exercise—less thinking and more writing!

Woman's Profile

Be open to the answers coming from within as you ask yourself each question. Give brief, spontaneous answers that describe how you feel.

1. When I first found out I was pregnant I felt:
   _____
   _____

2. Now I feel: _____
   _____
   _____

3. When I feel the baby move I feel: _____
   _____
   _____

4. In my dreams the baby has been: _____
   _____
   _____

   The birth has been: _____
   _____
   _____

   Other vivid dreams: _____
   _____
   _____

5. I sometimes worry about the baby's health or perfection: _____
   _____
   _____

6. The thing I like best about being pregnant is:
   _____
   _____

7. The thing I like least about being pregnant is:
   _____
   _____

8. Right now I think my body is:_____
   _____
   _____

9. Early in my pregnancy my sexual feelings were:
   _____
   _____

10. Now our sex life is:_____
    _____
    _____

11. In childbirth, I feel that most women worry about: _____
    _____
    _____

12. The worst thing I could do during labor/birth would be to: _____
    _____
    _____

13. The biggest question/uncertainty I have about being a mother is: _____
    _____
    _____

14. The main way I would like to be different from my parents is: _____
    _____
    _____

15. The thing I like most about my partner is:
    _____
    _____

16. The thing I like least about my partner is:
    _____
    _____

17. The way this pregnancy has affected our relationship as a couple is: _____
    _____
    _____

When your partner has a few minutes, explain that you would like him to do this exercise. Ask him to write whatever first comes to him without stopping to analyze his responses. Tell him you'll be back in ten minutes: don't breathe down his neck the whole time!

Man's Profile

Be open to the answers coming from within you as you ask yourself each question. Give brief, spontaneous answers that describe the way you feel.

1. When I first found out we were expecting a baby, I felt: _____
   _____

2. Now I feel: _____
   _____

3. When I feel the baby move I feel: _____
   _____
   _____

4. I've had the following dreams about the baby or the birth: _____
   _____
   _____

5. The biggest fear I have about having a(nother) child is: _____
   _____

6. The biggest question/uncertainty I have about being a father is: _____
   _____
   _____

7. The thing I like best about my wife being pregnant is her: _____
   _____
   _____

8. The thing I like least about my wife being pregnant is her: _____
   _____
   _____

9. During this pregnancy, our sex life has: _____
   _____
   _____

The way I feel about this is: _____
_____
_____

10. The thing I feel most women worry about in childbirth is: _____
    _____
    _____

11. The thing that most concerns me about labor and birth is: _____
    _____
    _____

12. I think of my own father as: _____
    _____
    _____

13. The main way I would like to be different from my parents is: _____
    _____
    _____

14. The thing I like most about my partner is: ____
    _____
    _____

15. The thing I like most about my partner is: ____
    _____
    _____

16. The way this pregnancy has affected our relationship as a couple is: _____
    _____
    _____

Now talk to each other about your own reactions, or ask questions about each other's responses. In childbirth education classes we do not discuss this profile. It helps people get in touch with their own feelings, so they begin talking about things on the way home or in bed that night. People's intentions are good, and it is usually only a lack of communication that leads to trouble. For example, he may be working long hours to be a good provider and to enable moving to a larger home now that the baby is coming; she, on the other hand, could not care less about a new house, is feeling lonely and abandoned by his long hours at the office, and thinks he doesn't care about her and the pregnancy. Talking helps.

Images

When we take on certain roles in the game of life, we usually have a preconceived image of how that role is supposed to be played. These images may be from social expectations, from personal experience, or from fantasies. Today many roles are in transition, and this can lead to misunderstanding and unfulfillment.

Getting in touch with our images of roles helps in understanding our own behavior and that of others. Following is a list of some roles associated with childbirth and childcare. Write in some attributes you associate with these roles and have your partner do the same, then compare and discuss. Remember, some attributes are "built in" to the role, some are merely traditional, and some are learned by playing the role. We as persons are not the roles we play, and we can often rewrite the roles if it seems desirable.

Pregnant women are: _____

_____

Mothers are: _____

_____

Fathers are: _____

_____

Parents are: _____

_____

Children are: _____

_____

Babies are: _____

_____

Grandparents are: _____

_____

Doctors are: _____

_____

Midwives are: _____

_____

Babysitters are: _____

_____

WORDS

Words and writing scare me sometimes
like the fear of some tribespeople
that a photograph will steal their human soul.

It's true,
when stark lines drawn on paper
and etched into our minds
are given the power to define
freeze
and confine.

Before you file me under
Terra-of-a-certain-kind
I may have transmuted my self into

Butterfly
Whore or Bitch
Whiff of Cinnamon
Potential Enemy
and back
to Terra-the-way-you-thought
 or maybe not.

Terra

Keeping a Journal

Keeping a journal can be especially useful for staying in touch with what you are feeling during your pregnancy and postpartum. It is useful as an emotional outlet, a private voice, a creative expression, a reality check, a memory refresher, a record of changes you go through, and a way to see patterns in your feelings over an extended period of time. Here are some suggestions:

● Don't chastise yourself if you don't write every day. Instead, reward yourself with good feeling when you do write, thus avoiding guilt feelings that may turn you off to the whole process.
● Feel free to draw, write one word over and over, or do anything you please in your journal.
● Try different colors of ink to express moods.
● You may like giving your journal a name or identity. It may represent your alter ego, God, or a good friend.
● Be sure to write down the story of your birthing shortly after your baby comes; maternal amnesia may soon set in, precious details may be forgotten.

● Go back every so often and read old journals—from last year, last month, last week. See your changes and your consistencies.

● Have a special notebook or blank book just for your journal.

● You might want to write your affirmations, dreams, and goals in your journal for later reference.

Pregnant Dreams

Dreams can help uncover hidden feelings and fears during pregnancy. Most pregnant women have at least one or two dreams that stand out as strange or upsetting. They don't mean that your baby is going to be deformed or that you are going to give birth to a chipmunk! Work with dreams in stages, first remembering them, then interpreting them or letting them continue to work within you.

To remember your dreams more frequently, it is helpful to:

● Suggest to yourself before sleeping that you will remember your dreams when you awaken.

● Write down your dreams as soon as possible after you awaken. If you begin to look at the day ahead, the dream may vanish.

● Don't try to analyse your dreams before they are written down, or the mental activity may overcome your dream memories, just as a stronger radio station will drown out a weaker one.

● Feel your mood when you wake up and try to tap into the dream through your mood. Don't concentrate; rather, let it float to the surface of your consciousness by holding onto that waking mood.

Dream interpretation is possible for anyone; you needn't be a trained psychoanalyst. Dreams are made of symbols that are meaningful to the dreamer. To interpret puzzling symbols or parts of dreams, try brainstorming, writing down all associations that come to mind. Also explore any universal symbols, such as water indicating emotion. An excellent book is *The Dream Worlds of Pregnancy* by Eileen Stukane.[1] Don't be concerned if dreams seem frightening; remember they need to be interpreted. One study showed that women who frequently had anxiety dreams had shorter labors than those who had fewer such dreams. The researchers believed the women were actually coping with their anxieties in their dreams.[2]

Here are some examples of dreams Terra had during her pregnancy.

● *After complaining a few days about the discomfort of my abdomen stretching, I dreamed that I was throwing up my baby into the toilet. It cried, "Help me, Mommy!" as it went down the plumbing. This dream helped me to realize that my thankfulness could exceed my discomfort.*

● *I dreamed that I gave birth to a baby girl. She could talk immediately after her birth. She grew very, very quickly. By the time I got to try to breastfeed her, she was already four years old and had teeth. I told her she had to nurse, since I had planned to do so for the first six months, at least. She asked, "Is that good for me?" and I answered yes. I bent my own head down and showed her how to suck, and I playfully squirted milk at her. This dream encouraged me to learn more about breastfeeding.*

● *I dreamed that I gave birth to my baby and he was physically deformed. His arms and legs were translucent and flimsy, and his penis was on his side, instead of between his legs. I loved him immensely. He could talk to me. The love I felt was overwhelming. It reminded me of the love I once felt when I dreamed of walking in a dark, underground tunnel and saw a bright, white light that I knew was the true Christ consciousness. This dream helped me to realize that no matter what could be wrong with my baby, I would still love him or her.*

Rahima reports:

● *After having two children, I dreamed I was standing in line in a hospital to get new glasses when I went into labor. I went down to the basement, got into a bed, reached under the sheets and delivered the baby myself. It was exhilarating, and I walked out with my baby. The birth itself was a midwife's wish-fulfillment. The real power of the dream for me was that the baby was a girl. Through the dream I felt reconciliation with my son and the freedom to have either a boy or a girl should I become pregnant again.*

● *As a mother of three children I dreamed I was pregnant and delivered the baby myself. I was tremendously pleased and handed it to some friends so I could get cleaned up. When they gave it back to me, it was a kitten instead of a baby. I liked the kitten, but then I thought I should be upset because they hadn't given me back my baby. "But a kitten is easier to take care of," I said. My ambivalence toward increased motherhood is obvious.*

Write down one or more of your dreams here:

_____

_____

_____

_____

_____

_____

_____

_____

_____

What Are You Feeling About The Baby?

Draw a picture of your baby as you imagine him or her to be right now:

Do you think of your baby as being fully formed? As having fingers and toes, ability to hear, distinct personality characteristics? Do you have a nickname

you call him or her? Or do you think of the baby as being somewhat amorphous, kind of a round, un-formed shape? A study reported in *Birth and the Family Journal* showed that almost all women thought of their babies as less developed than they were, regardless of their stage of pregnancy.[3]

Did you know that by the end of the ninth week after fertilization, your baby resembles a miniature human being? Even though only one inch in length and weighing about one-fifth of an ounce, all the major organ systems have been formed. By the end of the third month, your baby can make a fist, open his mouth, purse his lips and frown. He has grown to 3 inches. By the time you feel your baby's movements in the fifth month, she is 12 inches in length, with eyebrows, eyelashes and hair. In the sixth month your baby can hear and respond to sounds and is sensitive to light and dark. The baby is much more sensitive in utero than has been previously thought, and Verny's book *The Secret Life of the Unborn Child*[4] or Nilsson's *A Child Is Born*[5] are exciting introductions to what your baby might be like.

Any ambivalent feelings about your baby are more likely feelings about being pregnant or the changes you will have to make in your life when you become a new mother. If you actually feel the presence of your baby, love and attachment will start to form. This is what can make miscarriage in the first few weeks or months so much more painful for the mother than for her friends or husband. A baby can be very real to the mother, even from the time of conception. But other times awareness of the baby can be veiled either through the mother's lack of awareness, her ambivalent emotions about being pregnant, or by the baby's not revealing itself. One baby who didn't reveal itself took an otherwise aware friend completely by surprise. She attributed her missing periods to other causes and was dumb-founded to learn she was five months pregnant—with her third child!

How Do You Feel About Being Pregnant?

Let's begin by considering your views of pregnancy before you conceived this baby. Did you have to "fight babies away," perhaps having one or more unwanted pregnancies as a teenager? Or did you subscribe to the idea, "One drop of sperm and you'll be pregnant," only to find that it took you many months of effort and finally giving up in order to conceive? Was having children something you always knew you would do and fell right into, or did you feel pressed for time as your "biological clock was running out" and the doctor referred to you as an "elderly primipara?" (Elderly, indeed!) Was this a planned pregnancy or one that caught you off guard?

Talk to a friend or your partner or write in your journal about your *fertility* and note your attitudes and feelings as they arise.

When did you first know you were pregnant? Was it in the moment of conception, or not for a while afterwards? Did you know before a pregnancy test was given, or did it come as a total surprise? The variations are endless. At one extreme, Rahima knew she would become pregnant and even knew the sex and the name of her child, then agonized for six months until she actually conceived. At the other end of the spectrum is another friend who discovered to her shock that she was four months pregnant—with her second child! How could the knowledge have been masked from her for so long? Perhaps it was your partner who first knew you were pregnant and you didn't believe him? Did you need a doctor or nurse to give you the news before you would really believe it? Did false results on pregnancy tests confuse what you knew or felt?

Talk or write about the events and your feelings surrounding the *conception* of this child and your knowledge of this pregnancy (include other pregnancies if applicable).

Ambivalence is a key to women's feelings about being pregnant, especially during the first several months. This means there is always a mixture of feelings. No matter how much a child is wanted, there are always some feelings such as "Why now?" or "Are we really ready to be parents?" And, at times when negative feelings can seem overwhelming and lead to decisions to let go of a child, there will always be regret.

When did you first know you were pregnant and how did you feel about it?

_____

_____

_____

What did the baby's father say when you told him? What were his feelings? How did this make you feel? Did you share your feelings with him?

_____

_____

_____

What did you feel when you thought about telling the following people?

Your mother/father _____

His mother/father: _____

Friend(s): _____

Your other children: _____

Your employer: _____

What were their reactions?

_____

_____

_____

How did their reactions make you feel?

_____

_____

_____

Accepting the pregnancy means saying yes to being a vehicle for new life and allowing all the changes in one's own life and body which that entails. It may be a very difficult task, sometimes measured against ending the pregnancy or putting the child up for adoption. For other women, those questions are not involved, and yet accepting the changes in one's life and body can still be very difficult. Rahima intentionally conceived her second child but was outraged to find her sexual energy disappearing just as she had begun to feel that her body was her own again (conception was only 13 months after the birth of her first child). Resistance to the pregnancy, with its accompanying morning sickness, went on for months. When she finally accepted the pregnancy, she had a wonderful last few weeks. Most women are less stubborn than Rahima and come to terms with being pregnant fairly early in their pregnancy. It makes for a much more enjoyable time!

Was it easy or difficult to come to terms with being pregnant? Sudden or gradual? Not an issue or a major dilemma? What was helpful for you in accepting the pregnancy?

_____

_____

_____

Has it been easy or difficult to accept the changes being pregnant has brought to your life?

_____

_____

_____

What things could help that are still unresolved?

_____

_____

_____

If you have many unresolved feelings, a conversation with your partner about your ambivalent or negative feelings could help. Is there anyone who can listen to you without being judgmental (e.g. making you feel like you want an abortion or are a terrible mother)? Many times women feel guilty about the negative feelings they have; but once the feelings are expressed, they tend to dissipate or move toward resolution much more easily.

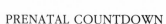

PRENATAL COUNTDOWN

Precious Parasite,
once, a fish, you swam
and grew on the waters of my ocean.
Now you are a creature
more akin to astronaut,
weightless in my inner space,
tethered to me, the Mother Ship
and not yet having walked on Earth or Moon.
(What do you dream?)

Soon you will be forced
to mold your head
to escape a tight situation.
And we will both be forced
to mold our minds
to form a new Relation Ship.
(What do I dream?)

Terra

How Do You Feel About Your Body?

Draw a picture of your pregnant body:

Complete the following sentences and circle those that apply:

Pregnant women look: _____

_____

_____

Pregnant women should/should not be seen at the beach or pool because: _____

_____

_____

I love to show my body at the beach or pool because: I feel so good/the baby likes the sun/I enjoy feeling free and expressive/I like everyone to know.

OR:

I would not show my body at the beach or pool because: I feel fat/I want to protect the baby/I like privacy/it's none of people's business/my husband would disapprove/it's not right.

Pregnancy used to be called *confinement,* a word which has fallen out of favor as Victorian attitudes toward sexuality have changed and women have stayed active and in the workplace during their pregnancies. The words for "pregnancy" and "embarrassment" are actually the same in Spanish. Imagine going around being embarrassed and showing it for nine months! In contrast, many women today wear maternity shirts that have "Baby" with an arrow, or "We should have danced all night!" emblazoned across the front. And pregnant women in bikinis are not at all uncommon on the nation's beaches. Our attitudes continue to change!

How did you feel about your body when you first began to show? Did you feel fat or delighted? Did you buy maternity clothes as soon as possible or avoid them for as long as possible? Any answer is correct! The fun thing is talking about it— not even trying to figure out *why,* just noting what you felt, and what you feel, and how it changes or stays the same. Feelings are a part of pregnancy. They don't make you into a bad or good person, they are just there to be noted as part of the tapestry of these nine months.

Breasts can become very touchy during pregnancy, both emotionally and physically. Swelling and tenderness require extra care and a pregnancy support bra. Women have many emotions associated with their breasts. They often have emotional pain from feeling they were too large or too small during adolescence. Pregnancy and lactation obviously make breasts larger, with accompanying joy or misgivings. We highly recommend the book *Breasts: Women Speak about Their Breasts and Their Lives* by Ayalah and Weinstock for further exploration.[6]

Women also tend to have a lot of emotional energy invested in their weight, and very few are free from the tyranny of the scales. Brought up as teenagers on the Madison Avenue ideals of thin, flat stomachs and high, full breasts, very few women match the ideal they set for themselves. They engage in a constant round of dieting and sporadic exercise in an attempt to change themselves. Many women are amazed to find that a feature their partner likes most about them is something they have always liked least.

Pregnancy changes body image and the cycle of dieting for better or for worse. As a woman's body goes through undeniable and sometimes irrevocable changes, her self-image, sexuality and body image are also called into question. This can be very freeing and the resulting acceptance of oneself can allow for a new emergence of sexuality. Being unable to stop the pounds from going on can free a woman from worrying about each half-pound she gains. *Or* doctors can impose a new tyranny of the scales on women who have never been concerned about their weight. "Mrs. Brown, you've already gained 25 pounds and I want you to limit yourself to half a pound a week from now on! You know there are dangers from too much weight gain!"

Weight gain in pregnancy is not dangerous per se; it is sudden weight gain from water retention that can signify a dangerous condition known as toxemia. Dr. Tom Brewer has shown that sufficient weight gain through good nutrition is important in *preventing* toxemia and other complications of pregnancy, as well as complications for the newborn. Limiting caloric or salt intake, or taking diuretics, are contraindicated during pregnancy. Thirty or even thirty-five pounds gained from eating nutritious food is good for both you and your baby, and you will be able to lose it after the baby comes.

For more specific recommendations about healthy eating during pregnancy, see *What Every Pregnant Woman Should Know* by Gail and Tom Brewer[7] or *Special Delivery* by Rahima Baldwin.

How did you feel about your body before becoming pregnant?

_____

_____

_____

What have been your feelings about weight gain during pregnancy?

_____

_____

_____

Do you feel full and fertile, or fat and dumpy?

_____

_____

_____

Many women are afraid of what their bodies will be like after having a baby. Just as having intercourse for the first time signifies a whole new phase of life and an entirely different relationship to one's body, so having a baby leaves nothing unchanged. Hips tend to be rounder, breasts fuller and lower, nipples larger, stomachs rounder. Women who do self-examination will notice that the cervix changes and the vaginal opening looks different. The pelvic floor muscles are more relaxed after birth, often making your insides feel like they are falling out; or shoulder stands cause the vagina to take in air and make strange noises. Internal health and vitality can be restored and maintained by exercising the pelvic floor muscles during pregnancy and postpartum as described in _Special Delivery_.

Stretch marks concern many women; the elasticity of the skin and the amount of stretching seem to be primary determining factors, but good nutrition and Vitamin E cream may help.

Most women are concerned about losing weight after the birth. Although this is naturally recommended, it's important not to be in too much of a hurry. You will be about the same size postpartum as you were at five months of pregnancy—don't torture yourself by trying to fit into prepregnancy clothes or by going on an immediate diet. Regaining your strength and maintaining adequate nutrition for breastfeeding must come first. The fact that breastfeeding burns an extra 1000 calories per day makes slow and steady weight loss quite possible if you eat nutritious foods and avoid those high in calories and low in everything else!

If you are breastfeeding, you should probably allow a year for your body to be really back in shape (although we need to remind you that it won't be exactly the same as it was). Remember also that breasts, hormones and menstrual cycles will be in an altered condition for the entire time of lactation.

Despite all of the above changes, many women find they are more comfortable with their bodies after having a baby. Somehow they "inhabit" them more and aren't as concerned with each half pound of weight! They move with more assurance and are more comfortable in their sexuality. Other women have a difficult time feeling that their body is theirs again, or feeling sexually attractive. In a society that honors the youthful images of Twiggy above images of fertility, our images of mature women's bodies often strike terror into a pregnant mother's soul. Rahima was amazed when her husband revealed that he was turned on by the round bellies of women who had given birth. She had always considered her "pooch" of fat unseemly. Who ever told us that men _value_ fertility? Who ever told them?

Many of our images of women's bodies come from impressions our mother's bodies made on us when we were very little, when breasts and stomachs seemed so enormous. Or we may retain images of ancient tribeswomen with sagging breasts from _National Geographic_. Although the authors haven't read any studies or comparisons in this area, we suspect that women feel much better about their bodies after having given birth than they think they will. But negative images of women still hinder us from being as sexual and as fulfilled as we could be, in all phases of our life cycle.

If you have already had a child, share your feelings about your body before you were pregnant and a year or more postpartum.

_____

_____

_____

_____

What were your images of women's bodies as you were growing up?

_____

_____

_____

What are you afraid will be different with your body after giving birth?

_____

_____

_____

Sexuality And Body Image

Pregnancy and birth are an intimate part of a woman's psycho-sexual life. A woman's feelings about her body and about being pregnant, as well as how she feels physically, greatly influence her sexual drive and desire for intercourse. Pregnancy and birth are also an important part of a couple's sexual life together. The medicalization and sterilization of birth have made many couples (as well as medical attendants) forget that giving birth is as intimate and important an act as making love. We once read a spoof called "High Risk Sex" which took the same attitude toward creating babies as is taken toward delivering them. The biting edge of the satire was obvious.

Marilyn Moran, in _Birth and the Dialogue of Love,_ discusses the similarity of pregnancy and birth to intercourse and orgasm.[8] Although we can't agree with her conclusion—that couples should birth entirely alone due to the intimate nature of birth—her quotes from birthing couples, doctors and anthropologists provide interesting food for thought. Chapter 7 of this book, "Pregnant Relationships," discusses ways of enhancing your sexual relationship during pregnancy, but in this chapter we are concerned with what you are experiencing now.

Are you one of the women whose sexuality and interest in making love disappeared the minute you became pregnant? Or did no longer having to worry about unwanted pregnancies release a burst of sexual energy between you and your partner that has been unequalled? Or did you find very little change in your sexual drive until your size in the last few months made intercourse less interesting? Elizabeth Bing and Libby Coleman, in _Making Love During Pregnancy,_[9] found from interviewing hundreds of women that four main patterns of interest in sex during pregnancy emerged, listed in order of frequency of response:

1. It increased throughout pregnancy
2. It increased in the middle trimester, but declined in the last.
3. It stayed the same throughout pregnancy
4. It declined throughout pregnancy.

This is an excellent book for you and your partner to read, and the beauty of their study is that no matter what you are experiencing, you're normal!

Draw a line showing your sexual desire during your last pregnancy.

Your pre-pregnant level			

1st trimester 2nd trimester 3rd trimester 1st three mos. after birth

Draw a line representing your sexuality during this pregnancy.

Your pre-pregnant level			

1st trimester 2nd trimester 3rd trimester 1st three mos. after birth

To better understand your feelings about your sexuality at this time, react to the following statements with an agree (+), disagree (−), or not sure (?). It may be helpful to write down your first reactions and then consider them more carefully. You may also find it interesting to do this survey at different times in your pregnancy and postpartum.

_____ 1. Sex is an important part of my identity.

_____ 2. My sexual needs are being met right now.

_____ 3. I could easily do without sex right now.

_____ 4. When I'm not sexually satisfied, I feel all right about masturbating.

_____ 5. Changes in our sex life have increased tension in our relationship.

_____ 6. It's easy for us to talk about what we want or like or dislike concerning sex.

_____ 7. My partner finds my body changes sexy and fascinating.

_____ 8. I'd rather that no one saw my pregnant body naked.

_____ 9. I feel like a blimp and as sexually attractive as one.

_____ 10. I'm jealous of women with flat tummies and trim derrieres.

_____ 11. I'm afraid that my partner will have an affair because he finds me sexually uninspiring.

_____ 12. It's been too long since I last had sex with my partner.

_____ 13. I'm worried that sex will affect my unborn child adversely.

_____ 14. I believe that pregnant women aren't supposed to be sexy.

_____ 15. I miss my power to attract men sexually.

_____ 16. I feel that there is a spectator present when we make love now, with the baby there.

_____ 17. I prefer satisfying my partner's sexual needs in ways other than with sexual intercourse.

_____ 18. Trying new positions for intercourse is exciting for us.

_____ 19. It seems as if I'm always sexually turned on lately.

_____ 20. Not having to think about birth control makes sex more enjoyable for me.

The last exercise may have brought up a few things about your relationship with your partner that you haven't discussed to the point of resolution. Pregnancy may involve changes in your sexuality as well as all other parts of your life. The im-portant thing is to communicate about them, so there can be understanding, respect and adaptation rather than blame and loneliness.

We have seen how body image can affect a woman's sexuality. Fears of being unattractive can certainly squelch sexual interaction. In a similar way, ideas that men have about pregnant women can influence how they respond to their pregnant wives. Fear of hurting the baby or causing a miscarriage can also be misinterpreted as his finding you unattractive.

What do you know about your partner's feelings and beliefs about pregnant women? What do you fear he feels about you? What do you know about his background and ideas? (In some cultures motherhood becomes associated with the Virgin Mary and consequently disconnected from sexuality. Nancy Friday, in _My Mother/My Self_, discusses women's collaboration through their own belief that "Mothers aren't sexual."[10])

What does your partner feel about sex and pregnant women?

_____

_____

_____

_____

What were his reactions to your changing body during your last pregnancy?

_____

_____

_____

_____

Is there any history of miscarriage or other medical problems that might be affecting your sexual relationship now?

_____

_____

_____

_____

How do you feel physically? Emotionally? Sexually?

_____

_____

_____

Are there other stresses your partner is having to deal with at work or in the family?

_____

_____

_____

Are your sexual drive or desire for intercourse fairly well-matched to your partner's at this time?

_____

_____

_____

Mismatched levels of sexual desire provide one of the most common areas of conflict in pregnancy. If the couple's desires are matched, or if one person is truly accepting of the other, there is little tension. But when one partner feels put upon, denied, unrecognized or undervalued, problems result. The first step is to communicate your feelings with one another and hear each other's responses. That in itself may lead to new information or understanding which can change the situation.

If communication alone doesn't resolve the dilemma, try to back off from intercourse and find other ways of giving pleasure to each other—touching, massage, kissing, foot rubs, and so forth. Explore ways to show that you care and to make the other person feel good. If the goal of intercourse/orgasm can be removed, even for one night or one week, both partners may be freed to feel the sexual energy that has been suppressed by negative emotions. A simple sharing of energy and touch can be very healing and is a definite improvement over a state of impasse. A man's willingness to forego climax for a time can lead to new levels of sharing, caring and excitement in relationships that have grown cloudy over the years or during the present pregnancy. Other suggestions for enhancing your sexual relationship are included in Chapter 7.

What Are You Feeling About Your Partner?

Pregnancy adds stress in a relationship. There can be increased closeness and sharing, but there can also be conflicts or problems due to misunderstanding or a lack of communication. One thing that can be out of synch is how involved each person is with the pregnancy. Because of the changes that go on in a woman's body from the moment of conception, she is often very aware of the pregnancy even in the first few months through symptoms such as nausea, fatigue or backache. While she is already deeply involved in coming to terms with being pregnant, the idea may barely be sinking in for her mate. Or she may be blissful while he's wrestling with the idea of increased responsibility, financial concerns, and what it means to become a father.

As the months go by, all of the talk about the baby, and the demands to be informed, attend childbirth classes, and "practice the breathing" sometimes make a man feel that he is out of place in a woman's world or is being supplanted in his wife's attention. Preparations for the baby, supplies, doctor's bills, perhaps planning to move to a larger home or apartment, all mean added financial responsibility that can strain emotions as well as the budget and also result in working longer hours or being more tired.

Men too must come to terms with being a parent. Emotions are brought up about their own childhoods and fathers as well as their desires for their own children. A new sense of fatherly responsibility may dawn suddenly, gradually, or not until after the baby is born.

A special section for single mothers follows, but for most readers your partner will be your main source of emotional support. So it is important to be in good communication, which means not only sharing feelings with one another, but also describing what _actions_ would make you feel differently. There is rarely a lack of love and caring between couples; more often there is a failure to understand what is important to the other person. Giving to your husband through frequent expressions of affection and taking time to be together as a couple are also important elements in maintaining a good relationship throughout pregnancy and having a new baby. Your relationship as a couple is the family foundation into which your baby will be born. It pays to put energy into maintaining it.

Trusting Your Partner

Trust is a necessary component of a working relationship. Trust means being able to count on someone. There are two aspects to trust: the ability to count on someone and the ability to be counted upon. Trust is a state of dynamic balance, with paranoia and blind faith being the chasms on either side.

1. **Name some areas where trust will be important to you during pregnancy, labor and parenthood (e.g. financial support, sexual fidelity, emotional support, coaching during childbirth).**

   _____

   _____

   _____

2. **Name your partner's strongest area of trustworthiness and his weakest. Be sure to talk with him about both of them.**

   _____

   _____

   _____

3. **Name areas in which you have had difficulty trusting your partner. Name areas where you can easily have faith in him.**

   _____

   _____

   _____

4. **Do you have any fearful fantasies in which your partner betrays your trust? Can you examine why? Can you discuss it with him?**

   _____

   _____

   _____

Communication Skills

Being able to communicate is essential for any enlivening relationship. In the case of a pregnant or parenting couple, it is the key to maintaining the relationship through the stress of changes and is essential for providing responsible and consistent childcare. Understanding that both listening and speaking are active parts of communicating is an important beginning to improved communications.

Some general tips

When speaking or listening to your partner, look at him. If he is shy, this may make him nervous, but couples can develop enough rapport to look each other in the eye when talking about important matters. Be aware of your body language when talking. Try to develop special times or situations when you can comfortably confide in each other (such as before you go to sleep at night or get up in the morning, or when you relax after dinner). If you are having difficulty finding time to talk, turn off the TV.

Active listening

This technique involves repeating the meaning of what the speaker just said to be sure that you got the intended message.

Example:

Alice (as she rolls away from Bob's caresses): "I am ready to go to sleep now.
   Bob: "You're too tired to make love now."
   Alice: "Yes, I don't want to do anything now except sleep."

Being clear with speech

Say what you want to say. Avoid hinting, which might not get the message across.

Example: Try saying,

   "Would you please open the window?" instead of
   "It sure is hot in here," if you want someone to open the window.

Say what you feel

Avoid name calling, which you might later regret.

Example:

   "I'm angry, you spilled that on my clean rug," rather than
   "You clumsy jerk!"

Be open and honest

Say what is true; avoid trying to smooth over how you feel or what you need to say. It is usually best to express something directly and immediately, rather than letting it simmer inside for days or years and then explode.

Example:

"I'm really sad you broke that. I hope you'll fix it," instead of
"Oh, it doesn't really matter, I guess," when it actually does.
"I felt hurt when you said that," instead of not saying anything.

Take responsibility

Own your own reactions, decisions and feelings.
"I'm angry at what you said," instead of
"You make me so mad."

Be kind with honesty

Don't use "honesty" as an excuse to be cruel.

Example:

Your partner is feeling down and you are irritated. Now is not the time to say,
"Did you know you have a big pimple on your chin?"

Try the following exercise with your partner. First, explain that you would like to try an exercise in communications skills and active listening together. You will take turns completing the following sentences. Decide who will go first. After one person speaks, the listener explains what he heard, using his own words. If the speaker is not satisfied that she has been heard correctly, she rephrases the statement. When the speaker feels the listener has heard correctly, she goes on to the next sentence. When one partner is finished, exchange roles and repeat the exercise.

1. Right now I feel . . .
2. When I think about the pregnancy, I feel . . .
3. When I think about labor and delivery . . .
4. When the baby moves . . .
5. When I think of myself as a mother/father . . .
6. When I think of you as a mother/father . . .
7. The best thing about this pregnancy has been . . .
8. The worst thing about this pregnancy has been . . .

9. I feel our relationship is . . .
10. After the baby is born our relationship will . . .
11. What I need most from you now is . . .
12. You help me most when you . . .
13. My favorite thing about you is . . .
14. My favorite thing about us is . . .

Negotiation

Negotiation is a way to settle disagreements in a systematic manner, so that everyone has a chance to express thoughts and feelings, and to agree to a common solution. It works best to discuss the process before a dispute arises. This particular process was developed by the Phoenix International Staff.[11]

Steps in negotiation:

1. Set a time to meet for negotiating a specific problem.
2. Set a location (neutral territory).
3. Define the problem.
4. Share the feelings each person has.
5. Show empathy for the other side.
6. Give specific examples of the problems so that both parties understand it.
7. Ask for feedback.
8. Suggest alternatives (the change desired, and if that doesn't get carried through, what the resulting alternative will be).
9. Set a time for re-evaluation of the situation, after a reasonable trial period.

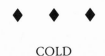

COLD

*In our winter frigidity
occasional warm words crackle and stiffen.
The dry cold rasps at our tender places.
When we touch, we stick, as to frozen glass,
and tear away each other's flesh when we part.*

*What once flowed between us crystallized into
solid separateness.*

We both beg for spring.

Terra

For Single Mothers

If you are having this baby without the support of the baby's father, you will need to put attention into creating a support system around you which can enable several different people to fill the roles which a husband might traditionally fill—confidant, labor support person, postpartum help, and so forth. Working with affirmations as described in Chapter 7 will help you to realize the support you deserve. In this chapter we will focus on your feelings.

Your family

What was their reaction to the news? How did you feel about their reactions? Given your relationship with your mother, what would you see her involvement being in this pregnancy? Is there another family member (a sister, for instance) with whom you are close?

The baby's father

Talk with someone, or write about your relationship with the baby's father and how it came to be at present. Is this a point of resolution, or are you still in doubt about his feelings and whether he will come through for you? What is his involvement with you? With the baby? Do you wish they were different? How? Try writing a letter to him, "I wish you were . . . I understand you . . . I feel . . . ." Now write another from a different viewpoint. Suggestions for helping resolve anger and loss can be found in Chapter 6, "Clearing the Past."

Along with any negative feelings you may have about him there is probably the opposite feeling of not wanting yourself, or anyone else, to feel negatively about him. After all, you are carrying his child, and who wants to feel negative about her baby's father? What would your feelings be if you had a baby boy? What if he looked like his father? These are all areas which, if relevant, should be cleared up as much as possible so your parenting relationship can begin with clarity. If what we have just discussed does not apply to you, explore what does!

Friends

What did your friends say? How did you feel about it? List friends who are especially supportive in various areas. Do you know any other single mothers with whom you can share experiences? Are there any single parents' organizations in your community? Call the United Way and ask them, or try asking the library or anyone who maintains a file of community support organizations. Call the major childbirth education groups in town and see if they have a single mothers' or new mothers' group.

Preparation for birth

Take a friend to childbirth preparation classes with you. Read *Special Delivery, Transformation Through Birth,* by Claudia Panuthos [12], and at least one book which focuses specifically on being a single parent.

Support Versus Need

Everyone has needs, and these needs increase during pregnancy and postpartum. Whether you are in a marriage relationship or a committed relationship or are a single mother, you deserve to feel loved and supported by God, the universe and the people around you. You will need to be able to accept help—something which is often hard for feminists, pioneer women and other super heroes to do! Of course, this does not mean you can give up responsibility and have people take care of you like a child. The opposite of "Super Mom" is a woman who manifests symptoms of illness or nervous disorders or presents her needs like a calling card— often with the justified fear that she might be imposing on others. Although such women are usually able to find someone (often a man) to "take care of them," the relationship is not furthering for either person. For a thought-provoking view of this phenomenon read *The Cinderella Complex* by Colette Dowling. [13]

Chapter 7 explores interdependence and independence and ways of being both supported and supportive throughout pregnancy and in other aspects of life. To end this chapter on "what you're feeling now," shade the squares from left to right until you are under the adjectives that best describe how supported you feel in the various areas of your life. You will end up with a picture (graph) of your current situation.

	Uusupported	Could Be Better	All Right	Improving	Supported
Your physical condition					
Your emotional condition					
Your relationship with your partner					
Your situation at work (if applicable)					
Your relations with other children (if applicable)					
Your financial situation					
Your living situation					

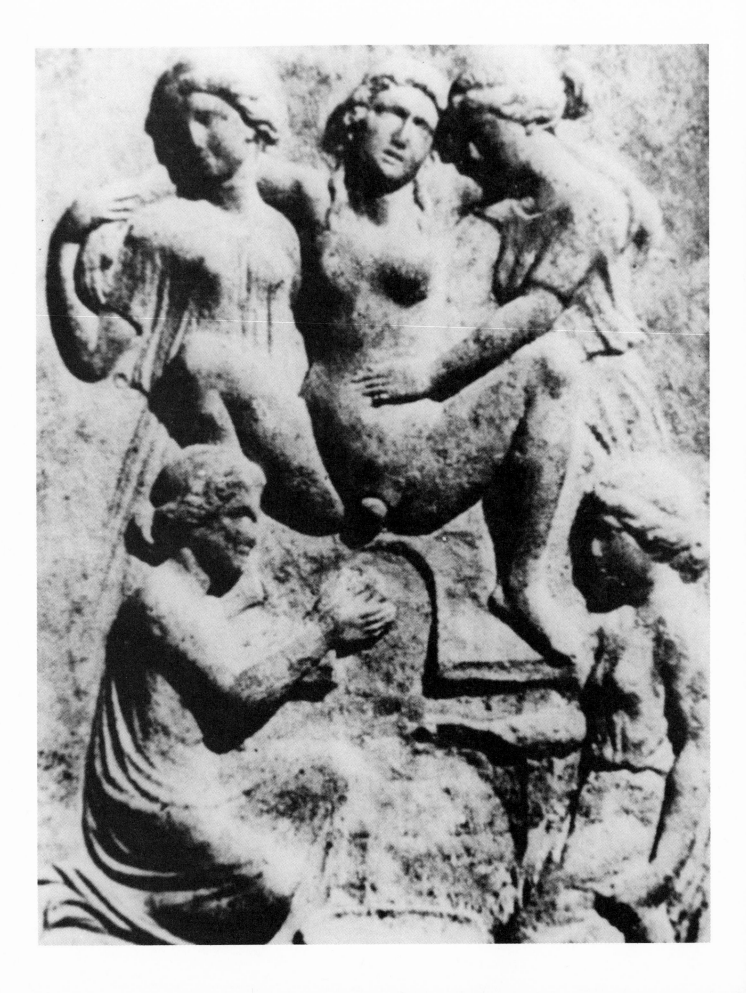

3
Birth:
Images and Reality

Giving birth is not an isolated event in a person's life. A woman births with both her mind and her body and participates in the attitudes toward childbearing of her culture and her family. Anthropologists' reports of women working in the fields, going to a sheltered spot to drop their babies without any "preparation" and then returning to work describe a kind of mythical natural childbirth that is nearly impossible for Western women. We are far too cerebral, and our twentieth-century consciousness intrudes between us and our instinctual selves. The fact that we question both how to birth and how to parent shows how awake our consciousness is. We must of necessity involve our minds in understanding what we do and create, for it is impossible to turn them off. Nor can we simply erase, or afford to ignore, our culture's view that giving birth is a dangerous and painful event requiring intervention and technology. Rather, we must consciously replace that view with new knowledge and new images if we are going to be able to reclaim our ability to birth with harmony of mind and body.

Our task is to integrate our minds and bodies, so we can give birth in a way that feels whole and nurturing—to ourselves as parents and to our babies as envoys of the future. We cannot go back to a "natural childbirth" in which we just let it happen. There must be knowledge of birth and an assumption of responsibility for our own health care and for decisions affecting ourselves and our children. There exists for us the exciting possibility of giving birth with full awareness, participating in the joy and exhilaration of working in harmony with the tremendous energy of creation. But it does not occur automatically or unconsciously. Rahima discovered in Mexico that the village women who were giving birth at home, in conditions that could only be called "natural," dealt with birth by gripping the mattress or by calling on the Virgin Mary. Whatever their personal style, they managed because it was women's lot and one had to get through it. Their affluent sisters in the big cities went to hospitals for anesthesia and would not think of birthing at home like the peasants. The possibility of birthing with a new awareness had not yet come to these women.

The potential for conscious birthing can exist independently of the place of birth, although some places require more watchfulness than others. It can occur in a labor lasting three hours or in one that goes on for three days. What precisely is it? Cohen and Estner call it "purebirth";[1] Panuthos calls it "positive birthing."[2] Let us just say that it is actively giving birth in an environment which is woman-centered and child-centered, in which the cues are taken from the birthing woman while she experiences fully the sensations and emotions of new life coming into the world through her. She is not medicated, managed or manipulated, but is supported with the knowledge, love and experience of her attendants (doctors, midwives, husband, other support people) to birth in a way which is safe, yet does not deny the intense physical, emotional and spiritual aspects of giving birth.

Birthing in this way is rare in today's culture. Cohen and Estner estimate that less than 5 percent of women in this country today experience "purebirth."[3] But it is accessible to all. However, it takes preparation, both to understand pregnancy and one's body and to find those attendants and the setting in which you can do the work of labor in your own way. The book work of understanding birth and the foot work of determining where and with whom you will give birth, are most effective when accompanied by the inner work of understanding your own emotions, ideas and conditioning. Familiarity with our own inner landscape can help free us from erroneous ideas or decisions that are not furthering to growth or birthing. By under-

standing the forces that have helped shape our concepts of the world we can begin to see patterns of behavior in which we may be trapped again and again and which always affect us adversely. That similar situations seem to keep happening to us over and over again is no accident.

Just recognizing our patterns of behavior and their sources can allow some of these nonproductive behaviors to fall away. Simply bringing them to consciousness or seeing the underlying assumptions that have held them in place can help release some nonproductive patterns as we realize our freedom to allow something different to happen. Other patterns are held tightly in place by trapped emotional energy from past incidents which have caused us pain; releasing some of these trapped emotions can help to free us in these areas. In other words, some patterns release effortlessly, while others require more work, and still others cling tenaciously or are like the rings of an onion—we think we've handled something only to find it coming up again in another variation.

The exercises in this book can help in clearing the underbrush of nonproductive images, ideas and emotional reactions about giving birth. This can leave us more free—to co-create what happens to us, to be more fully aligned with the will of God, to be in a higher and clearer state of being—whatever words from psychology or religion best describe the process for you.

In this chapter we consider the images of birth that come from society. Those we have gained from our families and from our experiences with sex, doctors, and previous births, along with possible ways of clearing them, will be considered in a later chapter. Being able to let go of the past can make us more free in the present to have nurturing and fulfilling experiences rather than reruns of bad movies.

Childbirth in America

The history of childbirth in America is fascinating and has been detailed in books such as *Lying In* by Richard and Dorothy Wertz.[4] Our Puritan ancestors drew their tradition from a Judeo-Christian heritage in which Eve was cursed with pain in childbirth as part of the Fall from Grace. The idea that the pain of childbirth was divine punishment for Original Sin was so strong that churchmen spoke out against the first use of anesthesia in childbirth by none other than Queen Victoria when giving birth to Prince Leopold. Early Pauline attitudes toward the flesh as wicked and separate from the spirit have not helped women to be in touch with their bodies or to have an integrated experience of giving birth.

The medicalization of childbirth in America lagged behind but later outstripped Europe's. The development of forceps in Britian by barber-surgeon Peter Chamberlain and his family in the early seventeenth century and the increasing tendency to call in physicians for difficult deliveries because they had such "instruments" led to the gradual decline of midwifery and the rise of physician-attended births. The widespread acceptance of general anesthesia and the drug scopolomine at the beginning of this century led upper-class women to give birth with physicians, who had the training to use these new "boons." Birth became more concentrated in hospitals as it became more complicated, and yet the majority of babies still were born at home in this country as late as 1940. The fate of homebirth in America was sealed by World War II, when the shortage of physicians required the centralization of birth in the hospitals.

In a vain effort to improve our statistics for perinatal mortality, doctors in the United States have tried to apply more and more technology to managing pregnancy and birth. The outcome has improved little over the years, for the United States still ranked twenty-third in infant deaths in 1987.[5] In contrast to this approach, studies have shown that attention applied to nutrition, prenatal care, and care by midwives or nurses can result in as good if not better outcomes than routine fetal monitoring and other "advances" which we are so hasty to adopt and export to other nations.

What has evolved in America, as expressed in medical texts, popular literature and the media, is the image of birth as a disease from which the pregnant woman needs to be saved through careful management by a specialized ob-gyn. The accompanying "just in case" philosophy has been the *iatrogenic* (medically induced) cause of the conditions it has been trying to prevent. "Just in case" you need a cesarean, we won't let you eat anything; "just in case" the baby isn't all right, we'll put on a fetal monitor that keeps you on your back and thus contributes to distress and longer labors. The total effect of such interventions in normal birth has been a major cause of the skyrocketing cesarean rate, which has reached 35 percent in some hospitals.

This medicalized view is so pervasive that many of us who had our babies at home ten to fifteen years ago had to ask and research such naive questions as, "Is it possible to have a baby without an

enema?" or "Is it possible to give birth without shaving the pubic hair?" We naturally assumed there was a good medical reason for the shave. When we discovered that studies in the 1950s had shown that shaving the hair actually *increases* the rate of infection, we good-naturedly assumed that the hospitals hadn't caught up with the studies. Now that another fifteen years have passed and such practices as shaves, enemas, and IV's are still routine in most hospitals, their credibility has begun to suffer!

The medicalized model of birth permeates our culture. The following sections consider images of birth from books, television, movies and other sources, and explore the effects they have had on our own pictures of birth.

Birth on the Big Screen

How a society feels about birth can be monitored by its portrayal in the media. Until about ten years ago, birth was never visible on the screen, but was portrayed by thunderstorms or other natural disasters indicative of its elemental and crisis nature. Or the ineptness of the standers-by was depicted through great fuss and flurry and such memorable lines as, "I ain't never birthed no babies, Miss Scarlett" from Melanie's labor in *Gone with the Wind*.

A decade ago television began presenting birth in documentary format. This provided powerful images of birth, for few people except nurses had ever actually seen a birth (until giving birth themselves). However, these documentaries have rarely provided models of a woman in anything but the customary hospital position and draping, and interventions such as IV, regional anesthesia and episiotomy have become so routine that they often pass as "natural" or "prepared" childbirth. Treatment of births in soap operas or other TV programs has been worse, usually emphasizing the heroics of the doctor or ambulance driver who saves the mother and baby in a highly dramatic situation.

The conventional medical views of birth so permeate our national consciousness that they even surfaced among the three- and four-year-olds in Rahima's preschool, who started playing "having a baby" after Christmas vacation and their experience with Mother Mary and the Baby Jesus. In charge was the traditional doctor (the oldest girl) saying, "Lie down here and we'll deliver your baby." One of the children even said, "If you want your baby sooner, we can cut it out for you." By this time Rahima was outraged at the futility of years and years of work as a childbirth activist and was biting her arm trying to keep quiet. The next day she tried nonchalantly to show one of the little girls that if she squatted, the baby would fall right out of her blouse. The girls looked at her as if she were from another planet. *They* all knew you went to the hospital, lay down, and the doctors did it. Obviously they were imitating what they had heard and seen, although several of the children had in fact been born at home. We had to ask ourselves, "What image does a child get of birth from films or slides?" You lie down, doctors and nurses do a lot of things to your bottom and hand you the baby. There you have it, birth in a nutshell.

What images of birth did *you* have from movies, books or television (prior to taking childbirth education classes)?

_____

_____

_____

What were your emotional reactions?

_____

_____

_____

Birth in Childbirth Education Classes

Childbirth education classes have tried heroically to prepare women for giving birth by replacing fears with knowledge that will help them actively work with contractions rather than feel like a victim of the birthing process. As dedicated childbirth educators ourselves, we share those goals, but we have periodically had to look at the images we were using in classes to see if they were really furthering to women. Since childbirth education classes provide very powerful images of birth, it is helpful to explore what they are and what expectations they create.

One of the most common images of birth conveyed by childbirth preparation classes is the model of an athletic event. The pregnant mother is seen to be "in training" and must practice with her "coach." At the birth itself, the coach is joined by the "cheerleaders" (nurses) who exhort the woman to go for it and PUSH while the doctor prepares to catch the baby and run with it like a football!

Such images present predominantly male models of childbirth. Dr. Robert Bradley, originator of the Bradley Method, presents us with another male model in his image of pushing the baby out like pistons in a car engine.[6] The model of the car is also used in many Lamaze classes through the images of first gear, second gear and third gear (levels of breathing).

Lamaze classes have also emphasized "painless childbirth," based on the book by that name by Dr. Fernand Lamaze.[7] While the work of Lamaze as it was brought to America has been invaluable, many women who have attempted painless childbirth have been disappointed or felt like failures when contractions still hurt. When Lamaze saw Russian women breathing and smiling in labor, perhaps birth only seemed painless in comparison to the screaming of untrained women, or maybe the American psyche is different from the French and the Russian. Perhaps the teaching has become so diluted that it does not sufficiently emphasize the condition/response training to the monatrice's voice that is at the core of the methods as Lamaze taught it. Whether for the above reasons or simply because of the compromises that had to be made with physicians to get "natural childbirth" into the hospitals at all, the percentage of women who attempt painless childbirth and end up with demerol, regional anesthesia or a cesarean has led many childbirth educators to shy away from speaking about "painless childbirth."

A desire to unite mind and body instead of using the mind to get away from sensation has led many childbirth educators to emphasize breathing through the sensations of contractions rather than trying to get above them. This change, together with dropping the term "painless childbirth" has accompanied a desire by women to reclaim the experience fully, including the painful and sexual aspects of giving birth if they are present.

At the other extreme from the Lamaze model in which the woman puffs and blows while her husband times contractions as she stares at an external "focal point" has been an impulse by some childbirth educators to encourage women to be expressive. They are encouraged to vocalize what they are experiencing, including grunting, moaning, singing, swearing or screaming. This together with the publicity about the benefits of squatting has resulted in an image of giving birth like the Earth Mother, grunting and howling. Such an image may be far too elemental and alien for the women sitting in class!

Another image of birth emphasizes that it is a sexual event, and suggests that couples kiss, hug, try nipple stimulation and "share the rushes of energy." Such an orgasmic image of giving birth may seem unattainable either because of hospital or personal constraints.

Childbirth educators have also perpetrated the image that *transition* (somewhere between 8 and 10 centimeters of dilation) exists, is horrendous, and makes you snap everyone's head off. Certainly there is often a short time of back-to-back contractions just before full dilation, but what a set-up that description is! On The Farm, an intentional community in Tennessee where the midwives encourage the women to be positive and to give to those around them, you can tell a woman in one of the videos is in "transition" because she is incredibly emotional, saying to her husband, "Oh I love you so much, I just love you so much!" The choices are ours.

Even the charts or birth-atlas drawings used in classes are nothing but models. They don't bear a lot of resemblance to the real organs. And traditional midwives in Mexican villages don't have those pictures before their minds' eyes when they palpate a baby, and yet they know what is happening. Rahima often wondered what images they did have.

Sometimes slides or videos of births shown in class can become powerful images to live up to. To the uninitiated, the woman in the film may look as if it's too easy; only a woman who has given birth will have any idea how hard she is working and will know what's behind the widening of her eyes in the middle of the contraction. Terra reports that she often mentioned in classes how her bag of waters broke while she was seated on the toilet, and one of the slides of her giving birth to her son Julien is of her in the bathroom. One of her students, while giving birth, insisted that her waters, too, be broken while she was seated on the toilet.

Given the wealth of images of birth that surround us, our task is to recognize that none of them adequately defines or exhausts the potential of birth. Perhaps their infinite variety can help to free us from any one fixed idea of giving birth and help us to realize our freedom to birth in the way that is right for us. We cannot control the energy of birth, but we can control our response to it by deciding to be open, relaxed, positive, noisy, grouchy, whatever. We don't need to behave in a certain way and we can accept ourselves and our births without self-judgment.

When Rahima first began teaching childbirth classes, she invited a couple to come back to the next series to share their experiences. The woman said, "I thought I would breathe and relax the way Rahima had taught us, but instead I crawled around on my hands and knees in the living room the whole time with my husband following behind me, trying to get me to breathe." For a moment Rahima was worried about the effect on her students, but then she realized that the woman felt completely good about herself and her birth, and that was a lesson more valuable than adherence to any techniques!

What we need is confidence in our bodies and our abilities to give birth. We need to reclaim the past by feeling our connection with all women who have given birth before us and know that our bodies know and are equal to the task at hand. Even dyed-in-the-wool cowards can give birth. (We know!) All new life comes to birth through the vessel of woman's body, and we participate in the timeless mystery of creation when we open ourselves to pregnancy and birth. We need to trust that power and trust ourselves, so that we can go where it will take us and open to it without fear.

The exciting possibility exists today to rediscover our relationship with birth. To help us do so, we need to look for or create feminine images of birthing that can speak to us in our hours of birth. Replacing male images of pistons and expulsion with feminine images of opening has been suggested by Kitzinger,[8] Peterson,[9] Baldwin,[10] among others. Midwives at The Farm in Tennessee encourage women to open to the "rushes" of energy.[11] British childbirth educator and anthropologist Sheila Kitzinger describes the vagina opening like a flower over the hard bud of the baby's head and tells of regions in India where an unopened flower is placed beside the laboring woman. Just as the flower opens during her labor, she knows that she, too is opening. Such feminine images with their connection to nature seem much more furthering than the man-made ones that dominate our births.

What images of birth did you have from your childbirth education classes?

_____

_____

_____

What was your instructor's attitude toward birth and pain?

_____

_____

_____

How did the women in the films look and behave?

_____

_____

_____

What were your reactions?

_____

_____

_____

_____

Birth on the Job

Those of you who have worked with birth as professionals may need to do extra work to clear up your attitudes toward your own birthing. Most of the births doctors and nurses witness involve high-risk situations or medically induced complications. Midwives and student midwives may have witnessed births that left them feeling afraid or powerless. The result is that health-care providers are often left with a fear of giving birth themselves. A pregnant woman was talking with Rahima about

her decision to have a spinal for her upcoming birth, and if that didn't work, she wanted general anesthesia for a cesarean. It came out in further exploration that she was terrified of the pain. As a teenage hospital volunteer, she had seen women moaning and screaming in labor. Through the exploration of other alternatives with women in the class, and the realization that anesthesia affects the baby and cesarean section is not an easy way out, she was able to lessen her fear. This enabled her to come up with a birth plan which had a greater chance of being fulfilling for her.

Sometimes nurses opt for giving birth in a birthing center or at home because they want attendants who have a more natural view of giving birth than medical students learn on their rotations in large teaching hospitals. But while wanting something "better," nurses often have an underlying belief in, and dependence on, technology. This can unconsciously lead them to need many interventions, whether they start out in the hospital or at home. If you have worked with birth as a doctor, nurse or midwife, look at your reactions to situations you have seen, your belief in the safety of birth and the place of medical technology, and your beliefs about complications, in order to be as clear as possible in your own pregnancy and choose the environment that will be best for you.

If you have been present at other peoples births, recount any that had a negative impact on you.

_____

_____

_____

_____

After each one, express the things you felt or wanted to say, but didn't.

_____

_____

_____

_____

What would you have felt if you had been in the woman's position?

_____

_____

_____

What was her experience of it (was she accepting, angry, grateful for being saved, in agony, etc.)?

_____

_____

_____

List at least five ways in which you are different from that woman and why that situation would not arise for you.

_____

_____

_____

_____

_____

Birth as a Sterile Event

Birth as commonly practiced in Western hospitals has become completely sterile—medically, emotionally and sexually. We have already discussed some aspects of the medicalization of birth. Although sterility is a good medical technique and is needed in an environment of sick people with attendants who go from patient to patient, a birthing woman does not have to be protected from herself, nor does the baby need to be protected from her. The sterile draping which is mandatory in a routine hospital delivery does more to disassociate the birth from the woman's sexual parts than it does to reduce infection. Women are told not to touch "the doctor's sterile field" thus created (in fact, women's hands are still strapped down in a few hospitals).

We would like to point out that the woman's nether region is neither the doctor's, nor is it sterile, since the vagina is so close to the anus. A woman should be able to birth in any position, even in the hospital, because it does not increase the risk of infection. In a birth center there is no sterile draping! What is the difference between one room and another down the hall? She should also be able to touch her baby's head before it is completely out or to touch her baby once it is born. The baby has natural immunity to the mother's germs both through the placenta and the colostrum that comes from breastfeeding. More neonatal infections come from the newborn nursery than from the parents.

Great progress has been made in the past twenty years to improve the emotional sterility of birth by encouraging the mother to be prepared for birth so she won't need to be knocked out. Allowing the husband to be present for the support and sharing he provides has also been a great help in changing the nature of giving birth. Indeed, it was Dr. Robert Bradley's recognition of and embarrassment at the emotional attachment women experienced with him at the time of birth that led to his conviction that they should be sharing the intense involvement of birth with their husbands, not with their obstetricians. His pioneering work with "husband-coached childbirth" helped change the American way of giving birth.

Further studies on the effects of emotional support on labor were done by Marshall Klaus and others in Guatemala. They showed that the presence of a *doula,* a woman companion during labor, significantly decreased the length of labor, the woman's perception of pain and the number of complications.[12] Yet most hospitals insist that a woman complete childbirth classes in order for anyone to be with her, and less than a quarter of the women birthing in America take such classes. Visit the maternity ward of any county hospital to see that the majority of women still birth alone and in fear and pain, attended only by occasional nurses who offer the best they can (usually painkillers).

Even when the emotional sterility of birth is ameliorated by the husband being "allowed" to be present, the sexual bareness or sterility of birth is ironic for an act that is the culmination of the sexual experience. This type of sterility results from male doctors being primary attendants in birth. In most other societies, men are not allowed to attend women in childbirth because of the private and sexual nature of giving birth. Indeed, even the husband is usually excluded in societies where women are attended by women. Since women have more experience with birth than a husband (who at most could be present only at his wife's births), women attendants in these cultures care for the laboring woman and maintain an image of birth as part of women's mysteries or women's work. They often feel that the husband should not see his wife in labor.

Men who are obstetricians and gynecologists have had to be businesslike with women patients, not getting emotionally involved, and somehow ignoring the fact that they are touching a woman in her most private and sensitive area. The extent to which women adjust to getting up on a table and spreading their legs was brought home to Rahima when she lived in England and had a pelvic exam lying on her side with legs *together* (the preferred British "Simm's position"). To the British it must have felt more discrete, but it felt "sneaky" to Rahima. In that moment she realized how much we as women deaden ourselves to the act of getting up on the table and spreading our legs to be worked on.

A British childbirth educator said she was amazed when she first saw standard American births. There was the baby coming out of this hole in the sheets! There was no woman involved, even though the mother was awake and aware. Her head was so far away, and she had become so dissociated from that part of her body, that there was no connection of the baby with the birthing woman.

Birth as a Rite of Passage

Anthropologists describe rituals which mark important transition points in life as *rites of passage*. These rites involve certain prescribed and inviolate actions which let the initiate and the society know that this person has left one role and entered another. At puberty, such rites mark the passage from girl to woman or from boy to man. Pregnancy and birth are a similar time of transition between woman/wife and mother.

Sheila Kitzinger drew upon her experience as both childbirth educator and cultural anthropologist to see the similarity between the procedures of normal hospital birth and the rituals other societies perform at puberty.[13] She explained how such hospital procedures perform the usual function of rituals by reinforcing the power of the institution to control both the staff and the patients. Most of the standard procedures of "normal birth" have no medical or scientific justification for their continued existence, as has been demonstrated in great detail by Cohen and Estner in *Silent Knife: Cesarean Prevention and Vaginal Birth After Cesarean*.[14] But the procedures' ritualistic function of maintaining the existing social order (i.e., the institution of hospital birth) is undeniable.

Kitzinger detailed six elements in a puberty ritual:

1. *Separation:* The young person is taken away from family and other support.
2. *Depersonalization:* The self-identity is obliterated, and the person is reduced to a childlike state. He or she is fed, petted, and allowed to make no decisions about when to eat, go to the bathroom, and so on.
3. *Ritual Cleansing:* A purging of the old self and ceremonial bathing occur.
4. *Inculcation of Fear:* Masks are often used; stigmata or signs of the changed state are made on the body (tattoos, circumcision); in fear and pain, the young person is given instructions on how to behave in the new adult state.
5. *Assessment:* Examination to see if the new state has been achieved.
6. *Celebration:* Return to the society as a new member of the adult group.

The parallels between the puberty rites and our own rites of passage in hospital birth include:

1. *Separation:* The birthing woman is housed in institutional rooms, surrounded by strangers (husbands are now "allowed" to be present if they know their appointed place and role in the drama).
2. *Depersonalization:* Clothes and personal belongings are removed; a hospital uniform is donned; a woman is unable to eat, move or go to the bathroom at will once the IV drip is hooked up. The shave desexes the woman, reducing her to a pre-puberty, infantile appearance.
3. *Ritual Cleansing:* Ye olde enema.
4. *Inculcation of Fear:* Attendants at birth are masked; fear and the need for control abound as birth is desexed and relegated to a hole in the sterile sheets controlled by the physician. Birth becomes a medical event performed on the body of woman, complete with deliberately inflicting injury of the genitals (episiotomy, or the cutting of the birth canal in 95 percent of births "to make it larger").

5. *Assessment:* Is she performing and progressing? Failure to keep up with the standard graphs is deemed cause for making the contractions stronger with drugs or using forceps or surgery to manually deliver the baby, even in the absence of any fetal distress.
6. *Celebration:* Some hospitals offer the couple a dinner of steak and champagne; others separate mother and baby and leave the woman feeling abandoned and anticlimactic.

In traditional hospital birth women are participants in rituals and procedures which maintain the institution at the cost of the individual. When will we as women stop giving our consent to such useless procedures and the male model of birth that seeks to regulate, tie down and control the energy of birth? The possibility exists to reclaim birth as the uniquely feminine act that it is, but in order to do so we must first change our own consciousness about what birth is and can be. We must realize that giving birth is part of our lives as women. It is a uniquely feminine act, one intimately affected by our images of our body and our emotions.

In London in 1982, 5000 women marched in protest to be able to move about during labor and to be the active giver of birth. Kitzinger reports that changes in hospital procedures finally followed. If we are going to give normal birth a chance to survive in this country, and more women a chance to experience it rather than the pain and frustration of the medical model of giving birth, perhaps we too must march to TAKE BACK BIRTH. We must realize that giving birth is connected with our sense of self-worth and with our rights and power as women. Birth has to do with love, sexual feelings and our most deeply held values. Birth is a celebration of life and must be reclaimed for ourselves and for the next generation. The sacrifices to technology that are made out of fear for the baby's safety are made in vain, because births in countries such as Sweden and Holland where most women birth with midwives have lower complication and neonatal death rates than does birth in America.[15]

But There Is Hope!

As we survey the co-option of childbirth by men, we need to avoid either complacency or blame. Men became involved with birth out of the highest ideals, and there are no villains or victims. Co-creation is real, and women cooperated in welcoming and asking for anesthesia, hospital deliveries and the latest technology. Because women were afraid of giving birth, wanted to be rid of the pain, and wanted what was ''best'' for their babies, they consented to being knocked out completely (in our mother's generation) and to a barrage of questionable procedures (in our own).

There has to be a better way, and there is. Tremendous progress has been made in the past twenty-five years through the efforts of organizations such as the International Childbirth Education Association (ICEA) in promoting family-centered maternity care, the American Society for Psychoprophylaxis in Obstetrics (ASPO, the Lamaze organization), and the American Academy for Husband-Coached Childbirth (Bradley Method) who have so dramatically changed the way women are able to give birth. Hospital procedures have changed greatly during this time, and will continue to do so.

The rise of birthing centers over the past fifteen years has demonstrated to hospital staffs that birth does not have to be the way it has always been within their hallowed halls. The incongruity of low-risk women being treated so differently from one room to the next can't help but bring continued change to standard hospital birth.

Knowledge of alternatives has been made known through organizations such as NAPSAC, Informed Homebirth, and others listed in the Appendix. And the growing acceptance of nurse midwives together with the legalization of lay midwifery in more states has made it possible for an increasing number of women to be attended by women who know and respect normal birth.

The baby has not been forgotten in all these changes! LeBoyer has increased awareness of the sensory openness of the newborn, and Klaus and Kennell have spearheaded changes which foster the bonding of parents with their children in the hospital.

Change keeps occurring. Whether you believe that changes are occurring because the children are demanding to be born in a different way or because economic necessity is forcing hospitals and doctors to listen to what women want, the power for change lies in our hands. We as women can and must reclaim giving birth for ourselves and then work to make these options more accessible for other birthing women. More and more possibilities are opening up for women to reclaim birth as their own rightful domain and to birth in the way that is best for them.

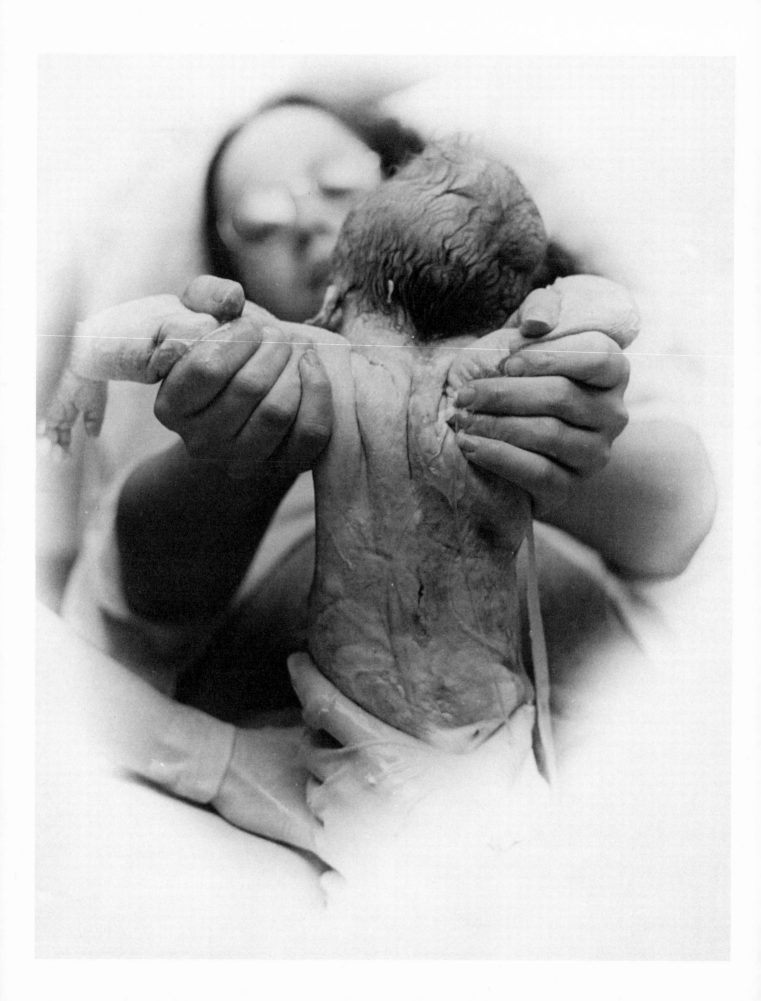

4
Birthing Renaissance

I t is happening. Women are taking back birth. The first steps came with being awake and aware. Women woke up to the fact that general anesthesia and hallucinogens like scopolomine were damaging babies and turning mothers into pieces of meat on which birth was performed. Because birth had devolved into the hands of male doctors, men had to play a major role in giving it back to women. Names like Grantly Dick-Read, Fernand Lamaze and Robert Bradley come readily to mind, but we recommend you read about the women in Edwards and Waldorf's book *Reclaiming Birth: History and Heroines of American Childbirth Reform.*[1]

As women began to give birth with dignity and joy, changes had to occur in hospital policy. Suddenly women were aware of what was going on and were able to participate actively and make their reactions and wishes known. Change in hospital policies has been further stimulated with the emergence of birth centers and the homebirth movement. And even greater changes are about to occur because of the success of the reforms over the past two decades. Hospitals feared and resisted the creation of birthing rooms, but now studies are showing that there is no good medical reason for emphasis on high-tech, mechanistic birth practices.

In close to a thousand free-standing and in-hospital birthing centers across the country, women are giving birth like normal human beings. They aren't prepped with a shave and enema. They can wear their own clothes and are able to have their husband and a labor assistant or other family members present. They are able to walk around during labor because they are not wired to a fetal monitor or a glucose drip. They are able to eat and drink as needed. They can deliver in the same room where they labor, and in any position on the bed or birthing chair. They are often attended by midwives or birth-center nurses who understand women and birth. One likes to think that they and their labors are treated more individually. And their babies are respected and left with them after birth.

At home women and couples have even more control over the environment, and over who is present. Midwives, who do almost all homebirths in this country, tend to see themselves as guardians of normal birth, and take their cues from the woman. Women are able to labor and deliver in their own home, experiencing the continuity of birth as a part of life. The homebirth movement has more than tripled in the past ten years and, although the percentages are still relatively small, homebirth is still on the leading edge in providing a model of normal birth.

Another such model is provided by The Farm, an intentional community in Tennessee. There self-trained midwives have assisted at more than 1200 births, 93 percent of which have been at home, while the rest have been in the local hospital or at their own Maternity Center. Maternal and fetal outcomes have been comparable to hospitals' statistics, but with a cesarean rate of 1.5 percent and forceps rate of 0.3 percent. The midwives' sensitivity to the energy of birth and work with touch to encourage relaxation provide a model of what birth can be when women work with heart and hands instead of medical interventions.

Numerous examples of women-centered birth come to us from abroad, where Dr. Kloosterman, Chief of ob/gyn at the University of Amsterdam Hospital, describes midwives' approach to birth in Holland as centering on the woman and her ability to give birth normally and without intervention. Or Dr. Michel Odent speaks of the clinic he has founded in Pithiviers, France, where women give birth in an environment that encourages them to be in touch with their bodies and their instinctive ability to give birth.

Odent, a surgeon who took over the clinic at Pithiviers, describes in *Birth Reborn* how he became interested in birth and began asking why the midwives did things a certain way.[2] With an attitude of openness and willingness to learn from women themselves, Odent and the midwives gradually developed birthing rooms which encourage women to go within themselves and follow their own best way of giving birth. Low lighting, soft colors and a low platform mattress avoid the usual associations of bed or delivery table. Women are committed to giving birth without drugs, because drugs upset the hormonal balance of spontaneous labor and delivery. During labor the women are not interrupted by conversation or frequent exams to chart their progress. Instead, an environment is created which encourages a woman to go beyond her rational mind and cultural conditioning and to open to the energy of birth, facilitated by optimal hormonal balance, just as in lovemaking. Odent states, "Indeed the harder we expect a labor to be, the more we pay attention to the *quality* of the atmosphere. Problems are the exception, even with those women whose past experiences would lead us to believe otherwise."[3]

We strongly recommend that you read Odent's book *Birth Reborn* and see his film by the same name.[4] One midwife irreverently commented that the film could be subtitled, "Male Obstetrician Rediscovers Women and Birth." But, unlike many of his colleagues, he *has* rediscovered them. He acknowledges not only women's ability to give birth, but also the appropriateness of women attending women in birth. He states: "The importance of midwives cannot be exaggerated. Regardless of particular obstetrical practices, more women have normal labors and births wherever midwives presently play a major role in childbirth, whether it be in Ireland, in The Netherlands, or here at Pithiviers. It is very important that midwives be women . . ."[5] He goes on to ask, "What is a man's proper role in a movement that seeks to return the childbirth experience to women? These are questions that trouble me. Presently I am seriously considering leaving obstetrics; this is at a time when male obstetricians would do well to retire progressively and restore childbirth to women."[6]

He sums up his work: "But Pithiviers is more than the sum of its parts. It represents an attitude, a belief in the instinctive potential of human beings and in the innate knowledge women bring to childbirth. Pithiviers affirms birth as a sexual experience, and encourages spontaneity and, above all, freedom . . . The introduction of freedom into an institution is neither an easy nor a trivial accomplishment. In fact, the concepts *freedom* and *institution* seem by definition incompatible. Yet, as our experience has shown, more can be done than is usually even attempted. Ideally, institutions can actually offer a sense of community."[7]

There are similar pockets of "rebirth" going on in hospitals in this country, where individual doctors have come to new understanding of birth. Scattered here and there in conventional hospital delivery rooms, women are squatting for breech births instead of having an automatic cesarean; women are delivering without stirrups; they are having twins in a relaxed and trusting atmosphere instead of an emergency, high-risk environment. Change continues to make its presence felt. More is possible than you may have thought!

What has characterized all of these births, uniting them and distinguishing them from birth as it is normally practiced? They have been women-centered and baby-centered, focusing on the mother and trusting in the normalcy of birth. Attendants have usually been women, who both understand birth and trust a woman's ability to give birth without needing to be managed or saved. The practices at such births have been much more sound physiologically than when a woman is on a delivery table with her feet in the stirrups or confined to the bed by a routine fetal monitor.

Have these changes in our way of birth been at the expense of the health and safety of mother or baby? On the contrary, statistics for perinatal mortality in birth centers, The Farm, homebirths, and Odent's clinic are better than those of surrounding hospitals.[8] There has been a marked decrease in the use of forceps and cesareans at these births, without any sacrifice in the well-being of the baby. For example, out of 1000 births at The Farm, there has been a cesarean rate of 1.5 percent. At Odent's clinic it is 6 to 7 percent, and he has a policy of *not* screening women to accept only low-risk pregnancies. The cesarean rate in America was 4.5 percent in 1976; it is now 18 to 20 percent. This suggests that cesareans are no longer being used simply as an emergency birth method to save the life of mother and child. Women have become so innured to the prevalence of cesareans that they don't realize what birth can be when it is respected rather than managed. The Farm and Odent provide us with two such glimpses. Compare the statistics in *Spiritual Midwifery* by The Farm Midwives[9] or *Birth Reborn* by Odent[10] with your own doctor's or hospital's.

Change is in the air and will accelerate. While birth continues to be an ordeal and a nightmare in many hospitals, women are waking up to what is happening and what is possible. The skyrocketing cesarean rate, the studies that show standard hospital procedures do not enhance birth or fetal outcome, the recognition of women's emotions following delivery are all contributing factors, but the change is really one of awareness. Critical mass has been reached, and it is suddenly perceived as too ridiculous and insupportable that birth be the way it is for most women. Women are demanding change. We have already seen women rally to take back birth in England. Odent writes, "The revolution so many of us are seeking will not be triggered by the professionals of obstetrics, or even by the medical profession overall . . . the most powerful movers of this revolution will be women themselves."[11]

And it is going to be the birth centers that hang the hospitals by the neck, for they will cause women to wake up to the inconsistencies of what is going on. Women are going to realize that, two doors down the hall, some women are giving birth like normal people, walking, laughing, squatting, eating, while *they* lie hooked up to IV's and fetal monitors and must give birth on a narrow delivery table with their legs in stirrups and draped with sterile green sheets. These women are going to start asking why. "Are the women in birth centers richer?" No. "Are there any medical distinctions between their pregnancies and mine?" Probably not, if you've been healthy and your baby is head down. "Is it just that one woman entered one door and one entered the other?" The simple answer is that some women asked for it. They demanded to be treated with respect for themselves, their babies, and their ability to birth. Soon all women will make that demand. Every woman should have the treatment women receive in a birth center, if not better. We don't mean that hospitals should rush out and buy wallpaper, potted plants or expensive, high-tech birthing chairs. We mean that women should be free to move about, to birth where and with whom they choose, and that their attendants should have an attitude of watchful attentiveness rather than a desire to control and manipulate.

The demand for change is increasing. Sheila Kitzinger states that changes are "coming from pressure by women to have the chance to give birth in their own way, in their own time, in an emotionally supportive setting, and with an uninhibited and joyous birth passion."[12] Why is it that Odent's work has been going on for twenty years and is only now receiving worldwide attention? Why is birth finally being accepted as a feminist issue in which there is an opportunity and need for decisive action? Why did hospitals fear and resist birth centers? The wedge of change has entered into birth, and the status quo cannot be maintained. Birth in this country will continue to change at an accelerated pace.

Reclaiming birth is part of women's taking responsibility for their bodies and their own health and well-being. The work of the feminist health clinics in offering women knowledge of their bodies and the possibility of self-examination of their cervixes has filtered into society to such an extent that a friend's doctor prescribed yogurt for her last yeast infection—a far cry from the days when Carol Downer and others at the Feminist Women's Health Center in Los Angeles were arrested for just such practices. Why was recommending yogurt practicing medicine when prescribing a cough drop for a sore throat wasn't? The answer—vaginal politics. Women are succeeding in reclaiming their bodies. Adrienne Rich ends her book, *Of Woman Born,* with the following vision:

> *The repossession by women of our own bodies will bring far more essential change to human society than the seizing of the means of production by workers. We need to imagine a world in which every woman is the presiding genius of her own body. In such a world women will truly create new life, bringing forth not only children (if and as we choose) but the visions, and the thinking necessary to sustain, console and alter human existence. Sexuality, politics, intelligence, power, motherhood, work, community, intimacy, will develop new meanings; thinking itself will be transformed. This is where we have to begin.*[13]

We don't need to change the institutions. We can let them figure out how to change themselves. All we have to do is stop giving our consent to the way women are treated in childbirth. If we say "Enough!" and mean it, everyone will start to scramble. The economics of an increasing surplus of obstetricians, combined with pressure from insurance companies to cut costs and government-imposed diagnostic-related groups, is going to help bring about the simplification of birth and the hiring of more and more midwives.

The economics is right. The signs are right. The realization is coming from a few practitioners and increasingly from women themselves. It is a change in consciousness in which we are all participating, regardless of age or race. The place of birth is not as important as the attitude toward birth, for any delivery room could be a birthing room if the woman could birth on a bed or mattress that didn't impede her position and she wasn't required to conform to so many protocols which wreak havoc with the birthing process. Similarly, home is no guarantee that your attendant will have a non-interventive attitude. Rahima still remembers with amazement that her homebirth doctor in 1973 had her birth on the dining-room table because he hadn't brought his portable delivery table! She also remembers that she didn't feel able to reach down and touch Faith while she was still partly inside, or to lift her up onto her stomach. She waited for someone to give the baby to her. But Rahima's realizing this was a sign of being free of it, of knowing that women can actively deliver their own babies and can be the first to touch their child if they so desire.

We need to support one another in bringing about continued changes in birthing. We need to support doctors and medical students who are daring to respect women and birth. We need to support the autonomy of nurse midwives and the practice of non-nurse midwifery in this country, because giving birth does not have any relationship to disease, and midwifery is not practicing medicine. We need to publicly recognize the home as a valid place for giving birth for those couples who choose it, and see that they have the support to which they are entitled. Now is not the time for anger or loss over what has been, but a time for action. It is a time to take back birth, to actively give birth with those attendants who share your understanding. And, if you are not pregnant, there is plenty to do in spreading the awareness that birth is creative and joyful and political, involving every woman's right to give birth in freedom and a loving environment.

Various Women's Dialogues with Birthing Energy (B.E.)

Women intuitively know that they are connected to all women who have given birth and to the energy that nurtures and sustains the universe. Here is what they have written. That knowledge can help give them the confidence they need to give birth with the full joy and power of their womanhood. We want to include here women's own words as they express their understanding of the energy of birth and their unique relationship to it.

> *Me: Birthing Energy, somehow you seem so near to me, a strong and guiding force, a channel to bring forth my child; effort combined with love and nature; many earthly and spiritual forces together to bring forth to the outside a living birth.*

The most blessed and continuously miraculous event that the Creator can bestow upon us. We (women) are but the home, the nest, and through us these blessings take place.

How better to seek a purpose or reason for life than to participate in the creation of one. Actually, Birthing Energy can be, if we are aware, the birth of ourselves as well.

Me: *Birthing Energy is Life Force at work. It is as if God has entered the woman's body and taken it over. It is holy and sacred, breaking down all defenses. I am in awe of the whole process. So perfect. Having a baby was like being close to death, to the edge, yet not dying, but giving new life. Like you have to approach death energy to give birth energy. It's the same thing. It hurts me to see such a holy passage be so abused as in the hospitals.*

After the birth I found a new respect for Life, and especially for women. I realized that it is the woman who carries the secret to life and felt that God chose woman because of her receptivity and non-aggressiveness. She does not raise up armies to kill one another, as men do. She is the keeper and nurturer. Birthing Energy is a privilege to be around. Something that happens every day and yet remains the most holy miracle that it is.

Me: *Why is it I never can get my mind and body to work together?*
B.E.: *You are afraid of me.*
Me: *Why do contractions have to be so hard?*
B.E.: *It's my way of releasing what has been held in nine months, a natural process.*
Me: *What will labor be like? I've heard frightening tales.*
B.E.: *It is the natural process of connecting with all women in space and time, which have been for centuries before you.*

Me: *Wow, you are pretty intense.*
B.E.: *Yes, I'm intense but I need not be overwhelming.*
Me: *But you're so powerful, so magical feeling, I feel as if I could get totally caught up in the sensation.*

B.E.: *It's okay to feel my power; you can't help that. I'm glad to be using you as a vessel. It's my pleasure, but this is the power of life. It's not yours to hold onto. You can only let me through you, and share in this power as the part of the continuum of life that you are.*
Me: *Thank God.*

Me: *Where do you come from?*
B.E.: *All women of the universe.*
Me: *Hey, how do I find you?*
B.E.: *Open up and talk to the sisters who have experienced, who also want to know how to find me.*
Me: *Will there be enough of you for me? Can you share your energy with all of us?*
B.E.: *I am unbounded and know no limits. I flow through all women. Just want me.*
Me: *When will I know it's you and how will I feel you? I'm afraid I'll miss the connection. The strong feelings I get—inexplicable to others and to myself—are they you?*
B.E.: *Yes.*

Me: (not pregnant): *Hello.*
B.E.: *Do you remember me?*
Me: *Yes.*
B.E.: *Have you learned?*
Me: *Yes.*
B.E.: *I am luminous, powerful, abound in all women. Pregnancy and labor bring the energy aura to a peak in all women. Nature responds to me. Life begins through me. I am latent in you now. Share with those who fear. Tell them I am not to be feared; only embraced, loved, stroked. What I bring is powerful, intense, and joyous. Ride above your body; let me work through you, through the children. Life and newness continue, renewed through me.*

Me: (not pregnant): *Hi and welcome, Birthing Energy.*
B.E.: *Nice to be here.*
Me: *Is it true that you are the truth of our being, the simplicity of life and death, that the truth of life is birthing? Your energy is so pure.*
B.E.: *Life has become too complicated. My energy is of simply truth. To love our-*

selves and body, to give birth freely and joyously, to welcome your child with warmth and love. Because birth is a spiritual event and also an intense moment of existence, it reminds one to be here now. We find truth over again. Simplify, live and grow.

Me: Thank you for being here.

B.E.: See you in the future.

◆

Me: Are you always present?

B.E.: As long as you have been, so have I. As long as you have seen, so have I. As long as the universe has been, so have I; and as long as you and I are one, so we are.

Me: How can we maintain and hold before us thy glorious vision?

B.E.: See through the eyes of a child the wonder and mystery of life. Feel the presence of never-ending creativity always growing and changing within you and reflected in all. Everywhere you look is the gentle caress of new life and the sacred and magical gift of life flowing through all. Re-experience the birth of your soul, and so you shall see the sunshine everywhere.

◆

Me: How can I know you?

B.E.: By knowing yourself.

Me: And be you?

B.E.: By being yourself.

Me: I don't know what to say.

B.E.: It is all within you.

Me: How can I be closest with you during the birth?

B.E.: By being close with yourself.

Me: What a blessing your freshness is.

B.E.: A reflection of yourself.

Me: What can I do to better facilitate my growth in birth?

B.E.: You can better facilitate your growth . . .

Me: Rest, relax, eat well, listen to my body. But what about all that I have to do?

B.E.: Drop that which is not important. Shed dead skin.

Me: I'm attached to a lot of stuff—and ways to deal with it.

B.E.: Be born fresh and new. That which is not, will not be.

Me: How may I always feel your presence?

B.E.: Always feel your own.

Me: Not my ego, but my soul, my true self, my essence.

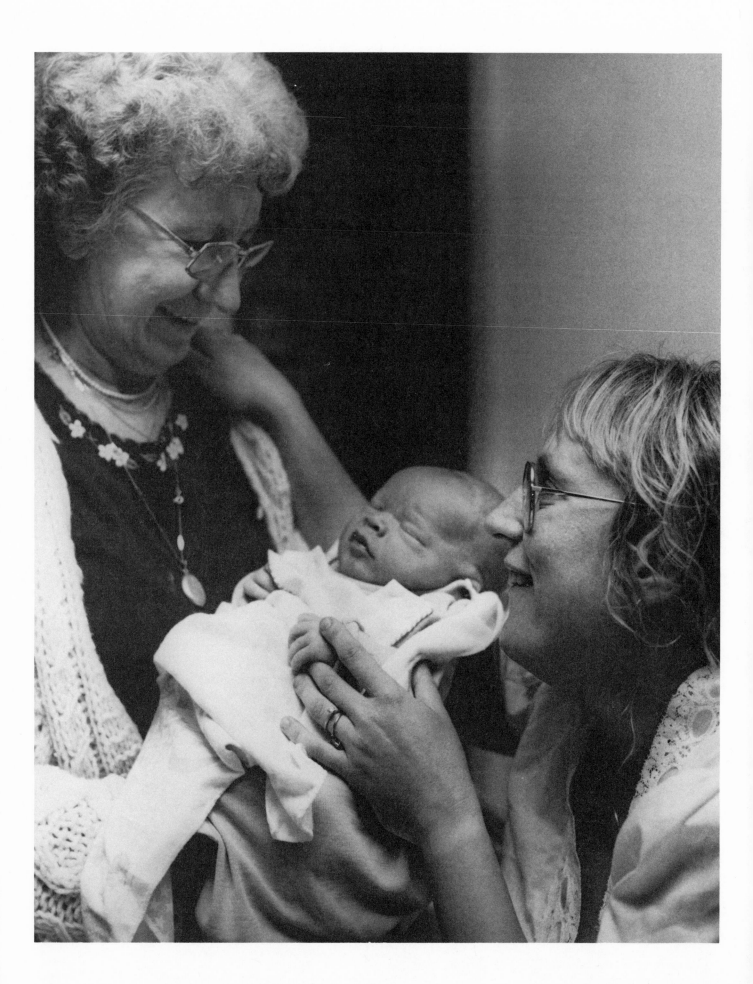

5
Recognizing
Your Roots

In the subtitle to *The People's Guide to Mexico* is the wonderful statement, "Wherever you go, there you are."[1] It is certainly true that you can't escape yourself! As women in childbirth we bring our complete selves to the experience: body, mind, emotions, habits, past experiences, lessons to be learned, and so on. Gayle Peterson states very clearly that a woman births as she lives, expressing this continuity of birth with the rest of a woman's life.[2]

To the extent that past experiences carry unresolved or trapped emotional energy, they tend to infringe upon the present. They convince us that what is happening now is just like what happened when we experienced loss, anger or hurt. Concluding "That's just how life is for me" after such painful situations also causes us to repeat the past rather than to create the present anew. To the extent that we can dismantle some of these considerations and free ourselves from their emotional charge, we can more freely respond to the present as it actually is.

In the next chapter, we talk about some techniques for dealing with trapped emotions and releasing unresolved inner conflict, but first let's look at some of the areas in a woman's personal history that can influence childbirth. As we do, you can note which ones are relevant to you for future work. Often just bringing past memories to mind (especially if you share them with a partner or friend) can go quite a way toward their resolution.

Birth in Your Family

As young children we imitate and emulate those around us. Because parents and siblings were then the most important people in our world, we unconsciously adopted their view of the world and imitated their intonations, gestures and stances, both physical and psychological. Even if we reject some aspects of their behavior or values when we are older, the similarities still resurface from time to time. As young children, we love our family and want to be a part of it. If that's the way the world is or that's the way things are for the women in our family, we unconsciously assume that they will be that way for us as well. Difficulties blamed on bone structure or a hereditarily small pelvis more often stem from unconscious agreement with what birth is like in one's family. Diagnosis of lack of progress or a disproportion between the baby's head and the mother's pelvis have very little to do with the bone size, as is attested to by mothers who have had vaginal births after cesareans (VBACs) and have often given birth naturally to babies who were much larger than their first cesarean babies.

By bringing to light some of the birth experiences of your family and making conscious some of the conclusions you may have come to, it is possible to take steps toward realizing your freedom and creating other options for this birth. At present just be aware of the assumptions about yourself and the world; in the next chapter we'll look at how to let go of unproductive ones and replace them with positive affirmations.

What were your mother's experiences in giving birth to you? To any brothers or sisters?

_____

_____

_____

_____

Did your mother talk about birth when you were a child? What message did she give you? If not, what messages did that give to you?

_____

_____

_____

_____

_____

What were your aunts' or sisters' experiences in giving birth? Are there conclusions that have been drawn about the women in your family?

_____

_____

_____

_____

_____

What does your mother feel about your ability to give birth?

_____

_____

_____

_____

The Weaker Sex

Women have traditionally been brought up to be out of touch with their bodies. They are taught not to touch their genitals, not to be overtly sexual, to keep their legs together, and to be restrained in their movement. Most women come to view their bodies as weak and ineffective. Even when they know that women can be athletes, they rarely have the experience themselves of climbing a mountain or running a marathon or doing hard physical labor day after day. It's no surprise that they wonder if they're going to survive the athletic event that birth is made out to be.

Times are changing, and more and more women are becoming involved with some kind of exercise, either outdoors or in the gym. Each experience changes one's self-image, body image and relationship with one's body. The first time Rahima fasted for 24 hours and didn't die, she had an entirely different view of the world and her body!

While it is helpful to be in good working relationship with one's body, it is not necessary to be an athlete to give birth. In fact, athletes don't necessarily have easier births. What is needed is confidence in one's body, endurance and ability to give birth. But nothing in our society gives us that. It is something we must come to ourselves. Events involving hard physical effort and even discomfort for some payoff—like the view from the top of a mountain or finishing a race—can provide models but there is no experience like birth itself to build confidence. This is one of the main reasons why second labors tend to be shorter. Certainly everything has stretched once before, but a woman's confidence that she can give birth, and her familiarity with its sensations, lead to much less resistance the second time around.

Discuss any experiences that have increased your confidence in your body's ability to work for you.

_____

_____

_____

_____

_____

Women and Need

One way of dealing with need is to be taken care of. This approach is ultimately dissatisfying, however, because it keeps a person in a state of weakness. While this can make the caretaker feel needed for a time, he will eventually grow tired of it, and she will resent him for cooperating in a relationship based on weakness.

At the other end of the spectrum is denying that any need exists. The stances of martyr or superwoman were probably learned at our mothers' knees. The martyr suffers silently under the yoke, not acknowledging her own feelings, and taking on more and more responsibility in a "poor me" manner. Superwoman charges ahead, doing more and more, while assuming herself to be an undying source of energy and comfort. Both take the route of denial: denying our physical or emotional needs, denying that it matters to us, denying that it's important to take care of ourselves so we can take care of others. Both roles are counter-productive and lead to burnout. If they go on long enough they can result in a woman becoming unable to tell if she needs something or what her needs are. Does that feel good? Do those shoes fit? How do you want to be touched? She doesn't know or is unable to say.

The question of how you want to be touched is important in labor, but women usually do not have much experience telling their mates what feels good. The extent to which women suffer in silence in lovemaking is staggering. Being afraid of hurting his feelings, being afraid of not communicating "right," feeling you don't deserve anything better—all are feelings that maintain the status quo and don't lead to a woman receiving what would be nourishing to her. In *Woman's Experience of Sex,* Sheila Kitzinger discusses the difficulties women have in communicating about sex with their partners. She suggests that self-confidence in sex is a matter of gradually getting more control about what you do and who you are. She suggests starting with something which is fairly easy and not too threatening to talk about, and then building on that success to talk about more difficult things. She suggests making a ladder of things you would like to say or talk about with your partner concerning sex, going from the least threatening to the nearly impossible. Then starting with the easiest situations, gradually work your way up.[3]

Is there something that your husband does in lovemaking that you just can't stand? When you think about telling him, what emotions come up?

_____

_____

_____

_____

Claudia Panuthos suggests in *Transformation Through Birth* that women's common practice of not going to the bathroom when they need to is indicative of the extent to which women deny their needs, both physical and emotional.[4] Does that make sense to you? Can you make an effort to be more in touch with your body?

_____

_____

_____

Often the martyr and superwoman go hand-in-hand in the same person. The superwoman takes on responsibilities under which the martyr then suffers. If both are present in yourself, imagine the two having a dialogue.

_____

_____

_____

_____

_____

_____

_____

_____

Women and Authority

It is difficult to create what we want when the authorities don't agree with or (worse yet) don't like what we're doing. From disapproval by parents, teachers, boyfriends, husbands, police and medical professionals, women develop a pattern of relating to authority that can decrease effectiveness and self-esteem.

One mode of reacting is to want or need to be saved. This can show itself by a woman manifesting physical symptoms or falling apart so that the other person will handle things. High drama and tense scenes often accompany this scenario. One woman's husband was a policeman, and when her homebirth ended up with screaming ambulances and the baby being born fine in the hospital parking lot, it seemed that we might be seeing *his* "movie," but she was certainly playing her part!

Another way a woman's relationship to authority can manifest is by her finding someone to whom she can give over all responsibility from the beginning. Dr. Jones, with his gray, wavy hair and kindly manner, is just what some women want when he says, "Now don't worry about that, Mrs. Edwards. I'll take care of everything." And he may take care of everything; the only difficulty is that this scenario breeds lawsuits. Wanting to be saved or being the savior is a dangerous game for both physicians and women to play, because giving up responsibility often leads to blaming others if everything doesn't go the way you want. Participating in decisions is a much more responsible path, because you're the ones who will have to live with the results of these decisions for the rest of your lives.

Fear of authority or feeling powerless can sometimes result in approaching medical personnel and institutions with such defensiveness that it's nearly impossible to be treated well. Fear attracts what is feared and maintains the role of victim. Gaining enough clarity that you can speak coherently without paranoia or belligerence helps you to relate to people in ways that encourage them to help you. Fear and frustration can leave you dissolving in a puddle of tears, even though you are trying to carry on a reasonable conversation. Such upsets usually come from past traumas and have little relation to the present situation until they recreate it in a negative way. Releasing past pain and increasing our ability not to feel threatened by authority figures work together to help make us more effective at getting what we want and need.

At a workshop for childbirth educators, Claudia Panuthos told of a woman in Boston who was in labor and fired the physician on call who came to attend her, for not treating her with proper respect. They sent another, and she fired him, too, because of his attitude. A third was also instantly dismissed for his remarks about her firing the other two, and they finally sent a fourth who apologized for how things were going and sat down with her to see what she needed. Rahima's gut reaction during this story was, "Oh my God, they'd kill me," and she realized that keeping her intention in the face of three disgruntled physicians felt nearly impossible to her. But this woman had been able to create what she wanted through her insistence on it.

We have seen that most routine hospital procedures surrounding childbirth are designed to keep women in the position of patients rather than actually increasing their, or their baby's, well-being. In the chapter on creating your own birth experience we discuss how to make a birth plan and have the kind of birth experience you want in a hospital setting. In the meantime, look at some of your patterns of responding to authority.

Do you usually feel powerless in situations with a doctor, dentist, or school principal? If so, how do you manage to get what you want? Remember a situation in which you got upset, and think of three alternate ways things could have unfolded.

_____

_____

_____

List three ways your ability to handle such charged situations has improved over the years.

_____

_____

_____

If you have experienced highly charged medical situations through previous hospital stays or previous births, read on in this chapter and the next for more concrete suggestions.

Your Gynecological History

A woman's gynecological history includes two major aspects—sexual and medical. Sexual attitudes grow out of childhood feelings about our bodies and from earlier encounters with sexual partners. The medical aspect arises from encounters (usually with men) in the medical arena.

An invaluable tool in looking at our development as women is _Woman's Experience of Sex_ by Sheila Kitzinger.[5] Kitzinger interviewed hundreds of women about all aspects of sexuality in the various phases of woman's life cycle. Rather than writing a scholarly analysis, she lets women talk about their own experiences. It is a very powerful and transforming book, and we cannot recommend it strongly enough. In the meantime, think about some of these aspects of your own growing up:

What attitudes prevailed in your home toward the human body, nakedness, genitals, and bodily functions?

_____

_____

_____

_____

Did you have any traumatic experiences as a child involving yeast or urinary infections, or sexual encounters?

_____

_____

_____

_____

How did you first find out about menstruation? What was your experience the first time you got your period? What attitudes do you carry toward menstruation? What has your menstrual and premenstrual history been?

_____

_____

_____

_____

_____

_____

What was your first experience of intercourse like? What did you feel? Are there any patterns that you have developed with lovers or your husband—suffering in silence, faking orgasm, experiencing pain, wishing he would only . . .?

_____

_____

_____

_____

_____

Describe your experience of your first pelvic exam and the circumstances surrounding it. Were there any painful incidents involving pelvic infections, IUDs, etc.?

_____

_____

_____

The above-mentioned events and attitudes help to shape our feelings about being women and are rich topics for consciousness-raising discussions. Experiences more directly relating to childbirth are usually more potent because the similarities with a present pregnancy are more obvious. If you have ever been pregnant before, and that pregnancy ended in a miscarriage, stillbirth, abortion, or a dissatisfying birth experience, your experience of grief and loss may still be unresolved and be impacting your present pregnancy.

The grief and frustration that surrounded a birth experience where a woman felt mistreated, powerless or out of control, can have lasting effects on her well-being, parenting and future births. Even if the baby is healthy and she feels she "shouldn't" be so upset, such painful memories can stay with a woman all her life. This is evident in asking older women about their birth experiences. The intense emotional quality of what they tell (positive or negative) testifies to how powerful the experience of giving birth is for a woman.

One in every three women who conceive each year in America experiences childbearing loss through miscarriage, stillbirth or abortion. Because of the extent of this experience, we will deal with loss and grief in detail in the next chapter. At this point, assess your own birthing history and note which areas will benefit by deeper exploration.

Did you ever have an abortion or abortions? How old were you? What were the circumstances and emotions surrounding the event?

_____

_____

_____

_____

_____

_____

_____

_____

_____

Did you ever experience the loss of a baby during pregnancy (miscarriage)? How many weeks or months pregnant were you? Was your grief respected and given adequate space?

_____

_____

_____

_____

_____

_____

_____

Did you ever experience a stillbirth or a baby who died shortly after birth? Were you able to see and hold the baby? Were the causes known? What has been your experience in the months and years following?

_____

_____

_____

_____

_____

_____

_____

_____

_____

Did you ever give birth to a baby who had birth defects or problems resulting from the birth? Do you fear something might be wrong with another child you would have?

_____

_____

_____

_____

_____

_____

_____

_____

_____

Did you ever experience the interruption of birthing processes by cesarean delivery? What were the circumstances and your feelings? What did you feel postpartum? What do you feel now?

_____

_____

_____

_____

_____

_____

_____

_____

Describe any previous "normal" births. What did you especially like? What would you do differently? How do you feel about yourself, your partner, your attendants?

_____

_____

_____

_____

_____

_____

_____

_____

_____

No one approaches birth with a "clean slate." As midwives we have seen women successfully and satisfyingly give birth who have had previous miscarriages, abortions, stillbirths, scopolmine (hallucinogenic anesthesia), and cesareans without their doing any visible inner work or outer counselling. On the other hand, we have also seen women's unresolved feelings cause complications and birthing outcomes that have been less than satisfying for them; some of these women later realized how their attitudes and emotions were denying them the kind of birth experience they wanted and went on to give birth another time with much more of a feeling of wholeness. One example of this was the birthing of a woman who had had a previous miscarriage, experienced spotting later in pregnancy, and feared a premature labor. Throughout her pregnancy this woman had worked at "holding in" this baby so it would come to term. When labor finally began, she had good contractions and all present expected the labor to progress quickly. However, for no apparent physical reason, the labor proceeded very slowly. Finally, Terra realized that perhaps she needed to give herself the permission to open up and let the baby out after all those fearful months of holding it back. After they talked briefly about this, the woman's labor progressed quickly and the baby was born shortly thereafter.

Removing blocks, resolving inner conflicts, opening, surrendering to the power of birth—all of these are processes which help a woman to birth with her full strength and joy. Loss and grieving can eventually be transformed into growth and acceptance, but that doesn't mean you might not still weep on your missing baby's birthday or feel grief at unpredictable moments. Once again, we aren't looking for women to be "clear" and without any inner emotions. In fact, the more comfortable you are in accepting your emotions and allowing them to be and to change, the more they will change and you will grow into increasing maturity and (dare we say) wisdom.

Birth touches each one of us so deeply and powerfully, because it involves life and death, creation, growth and transformation, both for the new being and for ourselves as men and women taking part in the drama.

Make a list of your attitudes toward birth or any other past experiences this chapter has brought up, if they seem to hold trapped emotional energy or if you fear that they might happen again. In the next chapter we discuss ways of clearing the past.

_____

_____

_____

_____

_____

_____

_____

_____

_____

_____

_____

_____

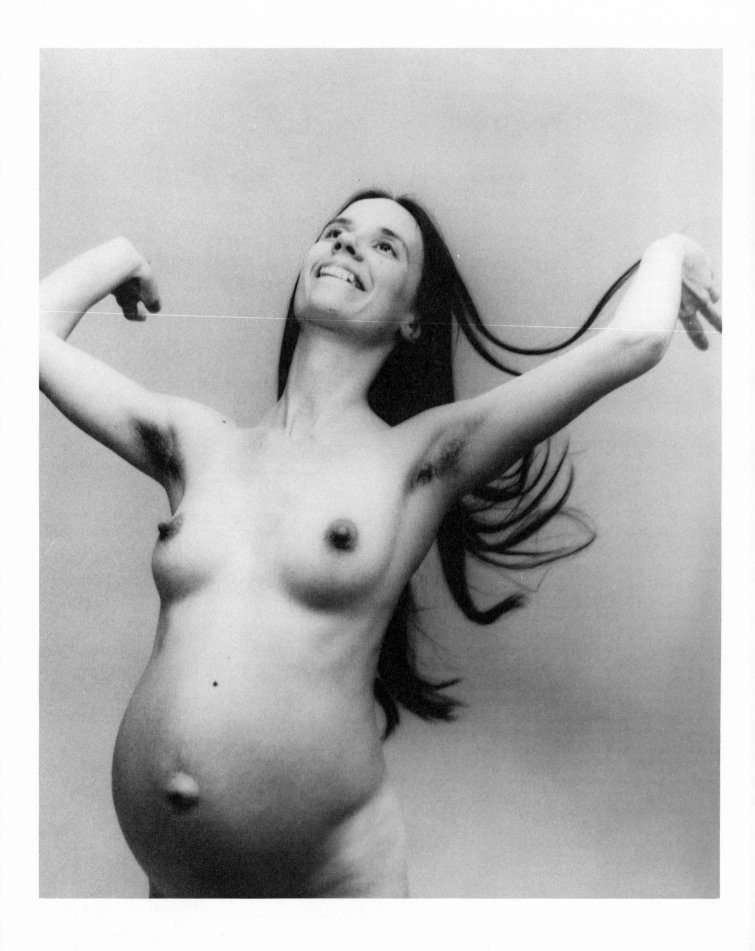

6 Becoming a Clear Channel for Birth

Many times our ability to experience the full joy and power of giving birth is hampered by past experiences. Perhaps this is our first pregnancy, but we find ourselves approaching birth with all of the distrust and fear that permeate our culture. Or perhaps a previous birth has left us feeling sad or angry if it ended in an unexpected cesarean or we felt powerless in our relationship to hospital staff or procedures. It can be very freeing to realize that it is possible to release emotions connected with past experiences and to discover and change the underlying decisions and conclusions about the world which may keep attracting us to situations that cause us pain.

Working with emotions doesn't make them go away. But it can help you to become a more energetic, flowing person who actualizes her potential to a much higher degree. For example, if you have experienced the death of a baby, nothing can or should make you into someone who has not had that experience. But if you are "stuck" in thinking every time the phone rings that it might be the hospital saying there had been some mixup, or if you're so angry at doctors that you're paralyzed at the thought of having another baby, emotional growth can lead you to greater freedom.

situations. We will explore many possibilities in the pages that follow. The techniques suggested here have been developed or used by us over the years in working with ourselves and with pregnant women. It's not necessary to be a psychologist to notice what works.

Tools You Can Use
The Written Word

Recounting an experience in writing can be helpful in bringing it up to consciousness. More growth takes place if you visualize the incident and experience the emotions that come up in you as you are writing. Keeping a journal can provide an interesting guide to your inner landscape, dreams and feelings.

Please find out as many details as possible about your own birth and any other labors and births you have had, including any miscarriages or abortions. Especially find out whether your children's births were complicated in any way. Write down the stories in your journal. Talk about them with your birth attendant.

The effects of writing are limited by the fact that everything usually remains internal. If there is no one with whom the writing is shared, a healing aspect of communication is denied. This can be remedied by writing letters. You don't even have to worry about mailing them—certainly not in the first several drafts! For example, visualize someone with whom you felt upset and tell them in a letter how their actions and words made you feel at your last birth. Tell the doctor or your mother or your husband just how you felt or still feel, about what happened. You may not wish to share this letter with them; the purpose is simply to let loose the stored anger, misunderstanding, and frustrations, so that you can begin to forgive. Forgiving someone else, or even acknowledging that it isn't yet possible for you to do so, is a very cleansing experience. Try this exercise in an area that is emotionally charged for you.

CLEANSING LETTER(s)

Dear _ _ _ _ _ _ _ _,

_____

_____

_____

_____

_____

_____

_____

_____

_____

_____

_____

_____

_____

_____

You may want to write the letter again as your emotions change in the writing. You may get to a version that you really do want to send or give to someone. Writing the things that have been brewing and festering within you and have remained unsaid can be very helpful, especially if it leads to dialogue and the clearing up of misunderstanding. But even if it elicits no response from the recipient, writing a letter can still have a positive effect in you.

Another possibility is to write down your feelings, then take all the pain contained in that experience and its memory and release it with the burning, burial or discarding of the letter.

Or try writing another dialogue with Birthing Energy. Think about your past experiences and ask any questions that come to mind or share your feelings with the energy of birth. Now's your chance! Here are some examples of what women have written:

B.E.: Hello, Marianne.

Me: Hi.

B.E.: I know you must have a lot to tell me.

Me: Well, I'll try to tell you what's been on my mind. I am still sorting it out. I am discovering the disappointments that I felt at Harmony's birth. It was not a long birth, and it was easy enough—no complaints there. I definitely felt you all around me for most of the labor. It felt very beautiful and serene at times. I am now realizing that the energy between Peter and me was not quite right.

B.E.: What do you mean? I felt a lot of love between the two of you.

Me: Since Margie (the midwife) didn't make it until the last 15 minutes, Peter didn't get to be the coach. He had to be the attendant for the most part . . .

B.E.: And you didn't like that?

Me: It makes me very sad when I think about it. It could have been a fuller experience for Peter and me if Margie would have come earlier. It did teach me, though, that I will do things differently next time.

◆

B.E.: Hi.

Me: How are you holding out?

B.E.: I'm here. I have been and will always be.

Me: Why did I feel that you were gone at times during my birthing?

B.E.: I was always there; the times you thought I was gone you may have been getting out of touch with me, but I was carrying you till you could get your feet back on the ground again. I never left you.

Me: Are you what I felt at the time of birth? That feeling of such elation?

B.E.: Exactly, the progress and love that has been about all during labor builds and intensifies as this new life makes its way into the world. This energy is what will "carry" the new person through hard times later.

◆

Me: Well, one year ago today (as a matter of fact almost to the minute) I first met you,

Birthing Energy. You seemed like such a gentle, friendly being those first few hours, as we took a three-mile walk, baked an oatmeal loaf, etc. Why didn't you warn me that you weren't showing your true colors? You hung around for a while thinking, "First I'll get her good and tired by making her laugh hysterically, get impossibly romantic and waste lots of energy, then we'll kick into third gear!"

When you started to really make me work, I wasn't prepared! At the time, exhausted and discouraged, I hated you and wished you were somewhere else—anywhere else but in me! I forgot why you were in me and that you were doing an excellent job of bringing me my wonderful baby!

B.E.: I needed to be tough and hard to handle so that you'd have an opportunity to learn about patience and strength. (Left incomplete when Rahima called "Time's up.")

Write your own dialogue with "Birthing Energy." Remember to write what comes to you, without thinking about it or judging.

Talking About It

The healing power of communication is well known. Its effectiveness lies behind the following funeral practice of an African tribe. If a woman loses her husband, for example, every person who comes to the funeral asks her how he died. She tells the whole story. The next person who asks obviously is aware of what went on, but she tells the whole story again. By the time she has done this for every person in the village, a tremendous amount of grieving and healing have taken place through the release and the necessity of looking at the events over and over again.

We have probably all had the experience of intense relief when we have found someone who will listen to us and not think we're crazy or "out of line" because of something we are feeling. Midwife Elizabeth Depperman Gilmore wrote a wonderful article called "Facing the Worst" in *Mothering*.[1] She described a woman who was terrified of dying in childbirth. Everyone discounted her fears or tried to reassure her. It wasn't until she encountered Elizabeth, who was willing to listen to her and help her work out what would happen if she *did* die (arrangements she would want to make for her family, and so forth), that she was able to make peace with the fear and go on to have a wonderful birth.

Just finding someone with whom you can talk can be of great help. If that person brings listening and counselling skills to the situation, even better. But it is possible to work effectively with a friend if you follow some simple guidelines. If you want to work in a concentrated way on releasing emotion connected with an incident such as a past birth or traumatic sexual experience, try to:

1. Agree that you are going to work together on an incident. Decide who will be doing the work and who will be doing the listening. The listener should acknowledge without judging or bringing her own experiences into the discussion. Things she realizes *she* needs to work on can be approached at a later time.

2. Choose someone whom you trust to be able to listen to you without judgment or personal confusion. The listener or witness holds the position of external reality while you go on your inner journey; it can be a friend, your partner, your midwife, someone with a background in growth work or a professional therapist. Try to choose someone who is not personally involved with the situation you are going to describe, because it requires a high degree of nonidentification for a mate or midwife to sit through your displeasure over their actions without reacting themselves.

   There is a similarity between midwifing and "psychic midwifing," or helping someone who is emotionally distraught or on a bad drug trip. At a birth, as with someone who is upset, by being there you are silently saying to the person, "I am here with you. It doesn't matter what happens, what you feel or where you go, I will still be here. And thus you can be here too." Providing this anchor point for a person is very important, especially in transition states. Perhaps it is also a function of the midwife for the entering soul, just as some hospice workers refer to themselves as "midwives" for the dying.

3. Set aside a time and place that is private and free from distractions. Make sure children are adequately taken care of; take the phone off the hook; put up "do not disturb" signs if necessary. A space in which it is possible to cry and make noise is also desirable. Be comfortable— choose a warm room with a bed or plenty of pillows on the carpet, and bring a box of tissues!

4. When you are ready to begin, close your eyes and remember where you were at the beginning of the incident—when labor began, or wherever you want to start. Go through and describe events in the present tense, letting yourself re-experience what you felt. Your listener should make quiet, acknowledging sounds, letting you experience what you are feeling and encouraging you to continue. She should not particularly draw attention to herself and the present moment while you are working on past incidents.

5. When you are finished, many options are available. You can go through it again; you can go through earlier similar incidents that may have been brought up. You can talk with your friend about that incident. You can do a visualization if she suggests one. You can take all the pain and attach it to an imaginary helium balloon and let it float up. You can pray and offer all your suffering up to God. There are no set formulas, so sensitivity and skill will help determine what to do next, just as they do in midwifery.

6. If your guide makes suggestions at this point, follow them only if they seem right to you. If you have much resistance to them, tell her so. Avoid taking out your emotional state on your friend through irritation with her. Thank her for listening. See how things move and change in the weeks ahead. Share with her any insights or further unfoldment you experience. If you feel you want a more guided approach than your friend is able to offer, seek out a professional therapist. A great deal can be done by working together if we dare to be there for one another, and remember who it is that does all the healing, and trust in that power.

Rahima would like to share two such cases. One involves a friend who had no experience in this kind of activity, but was willing to work with another new mother she met at a support group. The woman had given birth a few months before, but still hadn't healed from a tear in the rectal muscles caused by a forceps delivery. The friend listened to her recounting the birth, led her in visualizations of the area as healing and full of light, and was of tremendous help in the woman's releasing the psychic and physical pain that blocked the healing.

In another incident, Rahima found herself with a friend who was about to have a radical mastectomy for breast cancer. The woman seemed really out of touch with the magnitude of the surgery and the loss of the breast, so Rahima suggested they have a session together, but she had no idea what they would do. As they talked together, it came to Rahima to have the woman hold her breasts and talk to them. What came out was a tremendous story of emotional pain associated with having large breasts, blocking out sensation to and from them, and upsetting incidents involving boys and men and her breasts. Once she was able to be "in touch" with her breasts, she was able to reclaim them as part of her body and say good-bye to the one before she went into surgery the next day. She came through surgery with remarkably few side effects and her rapid healing time astonished the hospital staff.

These techniques are useful in a wide variety of incidents, many of which we would never anticipate. As a midwife, Rahima often used this process to review a birth in the first few days postpartum. By having the woman recount the labor and delivery in this way, Rahima could help her to integrate the experience, fill in missing facts or clarify confused areas, and see if there was anything that would benefit from further communication with her husband or the midwives.

Visualizations

Visualization is the use of the mind's eye. It is the kind of seeing we do when we dream, when our brain sees without any input from our physical senses. Visualization can be used in a receptive form, to become aware of intuitive knowledge, or in an active, creative form, to set energy into motion to achieve some physical, mental, or emotional goal.

Visualizations are perhaps easier and more effective when someone is present to lead you through them. But they can be done on your own, especially once you have the idea. Try the following exercises to sharpen your visualization skills:

1. Close your eyes and get into a relaxed state.

2. Imagine a Magic Screen appears when you want it. It may be like a large TV screen, a movie screen, a window, a blank piece of paper, or whatever suits your imagination. This screen will always appear in your mind's eye when you want it. It can tune in on the future, the past, the present, near or far, imagination or reality. It

can talk to you, and you can create on it what you will.

3. Now, see yourself on your Magic Screen, dressed in a costume which reflects your present feelings about yourself. Observe what this costume is, without judging it or wishing it to be different.

4. Now, change your costume to one you prefer, if you do not enjoy the one you saw. Surround your image with golden light of health and prosperity.

5. Say goodbye to your image, and to your Magic Screen, and gently bring yourself to your normal, alert state, feeling refreshed, as though you had just taken a long, peaceful sleep.

The Magic Screen is a symbol of your ability to tune in to the intuitive and creative powers we all possess, but may not yet have learned to use at will. Symbolic language taps into a more primitive level of thinking and avoids interference by our habitual thought patterns and random mental "noise."

Seeing yourself in Step 3 is a passive process, allowing the unconscious mind to project knowledge it has in a symbolic form. Changing what you see in Step 4 is an active process, aiming to change outer conditions by focusing your inner energy on a desired result.

When tuning in on receptive intuition, it is very important to remain emotionally detached. This is possible by remaining completely relaxed.

Some Helpful Hints about Passive Visualization

● Use visualization images to: help solve a problem; locate an illness; find a lost object; hear what your unborn or newborn baby wishes to tell you; or get inner feedback on an important decision.
● To answer a question, it may be helpful to visualize yourself meeting a guide, whom you may ask about the needed information; or see yourself opening a door or box, which contains a symbol of what you wish to know.
● To tune in on a specific person, it helps to visualize her or him as totally as possible, while holding your mind in an open and nonjudgmental state.

Hints on Active Visualization

● Active visualizations can be reinforced by drawing or painting a picture of the image projected. The

use of affirmations, which we will discuss, also adds psychic energy to the situation.
● Colors can be useful.
Associations Terra uses are:

> Golden orange: vitality, prosperity
> Green: peace, safe in Mother's arms, growth
> Yellow: love
> Red: creativity, activity, passion
> Purple: rulership, generosity
> Blue: protection, discipline, organization

● If you have an illness or problem of pregnancy: after dealing with it on a physical level, see yourself removing it by exhaling it with each outbreath. You can do the same if your child is ill.
● Always use positive images. See what you want rather than what you fear or wish to change.
● Practice using all the senses of your mind. You could visualize, smell, touch, taste and eat an entire meal in your "mind's eye." This kind of practice will also sharpen your appreciation of all that you sense physically.

When projecting a creative image, it is helpful to feel as much love, desire, power and confidence as possible. It is necessary to do everything possible on the material level to help bring about the desired result, as well as attuning the mind with positive imagery. For example, it is useful to envision yourself having a healthy baby; but unless you also eat nutritiously, exercise, relax, refrain from drugs, coffee, and alcohol, and prepare yourself for the birth, you are asking too much of your psychic energy!

The literature on visualization is extensive, and it has come to the attention of the medical community through work with cancer patients as described by Carl Simonton and others. That it is not only possible to release emotional blocks through visualization but to affect the physiology of the body is attested to by the many terminally ill patients who have recovered through visualization when traditional medicine has abandoned them.[2]

To use active visualization for work with clearing past traumas, begin with a relaxation exercise. This is incorporated into most guided visualizations, or you can do it yourself. Simply notice various parts of your body and release any tension, while imagining yourself in a relaxing setting such as the mountains or a deserted beach. You don't have to be able to visualize actual pictures to be effective. When you are deeply relaxed, do the kind of visualization

that is appropriate for the incident you are working on. Here are some suggestions:

● For a history of pelvic or reproductive disorders which you have had treated medically, release emotion by going through the incidents relating to that problem, beginning with most recent and working back to earlier and earlier ones. Then picture your uterus and vagina radiating light and health. See it as a creative power, not only in childbirth but in sexuality and all forms of creativity. If you have trouble arriving at that point, see if there are any messages the area would like to give you about what it needs or what you need to do. If you encounter any dark spots in the glowing light, allow them to expand until they gradually lighten (this may require repetitions). You might want to do such a visualization once a day, or even several times a day. These techniques of dialogue and imagining the organs healthy and working properly can be applied to any part of the body.
● In the case of painful intercourse after a birth or an episiotomy that won't heal, first go through the events and release the physical and emotional pain associated with the injury. Then visualize the area full of healing light, good circulation and healthy tissue. This can also help with the healing of a cesarean scar, especially with the laying on of hands to focus energy in the area. Release the pain of trapped energy and trauma through your helper's hand, and focus healing energy there.
● In the case of an abortion, relive and express the feelings surrounding the decision and the experience itself. Then imagine the spirit or soul that was to be your child. If you cannot imagine it directly, visualize walking along a path and encountering a young child. Say the things that you want or wanted to say. See if that being has anything to say to you. Is there forgiveness?
● Do a similar visualization in the case of a baby who had died or been given up for adoption. Express your unsaid feelings to this being. See if he or she has any messages or gifts for you.
● Many powerful visualizations can be found in *Ended Beginnings* by Panuthos and Romeo.[3]
● Once you have released much of the emotional holding power of a traumatic labor and delivery, visualize one in which everything goes smoothly. One such example can be found here in Chapter 8. If someone is leading you in visualizations, she can work especially with images that counterbalance your fears (your labor not being strong enough; the baby's head not fitting through your pelvis, etc.). Many images for specific difficulties can be found in *Birthing Normally* by Peterson.[4]

Decisions and Affirmations

Sometimes in the course of clearing or visualizing techniques, a person will understand why something happened and realize there is no further need to repeat it. Such a release is wonderful to experience or even to watch in someone else. It is another step in releasing oneself from bondage and indeed feels really free.

Sometimes this coming to a new realization feels like waking up; sometimes it has the quality of making a decision that you aren't going to be confused anymore. But it is very different from just making such a statement or from wishful thinking. With these, our habit patterns usually trip us up; whereas in this case some higher, more clear and free part of ourselves has come into action and lets its influence be felt in our lives.

Have you ever had any experiences like this? Does what we have described make sense to you?

_____

_____

_____

_____

People who have undergone such releases through the technique of Rebirthing developed by Leonard Orr[5] have reported seeing and releasing conclusions they drew about life based on the process of birth itself (for example, "The world is a cold place"; "It's a struggle to survive"; or "I have to work hard for everything").

If the experience of releasing a negative decision has not yet occurred, we can help the process by replacing the "negative tapes" which play in our heads and are fulfilled in our lives by more positive, affirming ones. These affirmations both carry the power of suggestion and have the same self-fulfilling character that our negative ideas have. For example, a mother who ended up with a cesarean birth worked hard and made the best decisions for herself and her baby. If she is feeling anything contrary to that, she could try affirmations like "My body is strong and knows how to give birth" or "I deserve to give birth with caring and loving people."

Such positive statements are effective because they work on many different levels. They operate on the psychic principle that "like attracts like"— positive thoughts have the same (or even more) power to be self-fulfilling as negative ones. They create a receptivity that can then be more easily fulfilled in the outside world. It requires less for the good to get through to you if you are oriented toward it and not putting lots of obstacles in the way! Affirmations also help you to understand yourself by seeing what negative reactions and other emotions come up as you repeat one of them. These responses will change over time as you continue to repeat the affirmation.

An affirmation can be repeated out loud, silently, or written over and over again. By jotting down any negative reactions that come up while doing your repetitions, more specific affirmations (and actions) can be created to deal with them. The next chapter contains examples of affirmations that pertain to pregnancy, birth and parenting. Experiment with making up some of your own as antidotes to negativity left over from past experiences.

Unconscious Release

We have discussed several ways of making conscious decisions or using statements to help release the negative patterns that keep us unfree. This release can also happen on an unconscious level, especially once we start orienting ourselves toward it. This happens, in fact, on a higher level, and is unconscious only in the sense that we aren't normally aware of it and cannot control how and when healing will come to us.

Sometimes the release we are seeking can happen in our sleep, because, just as our body is nourished in sleep, our deeper selves also receive nourishment from the spiritual world when we sleep. This is why inspiration, solutions to problems, and things we have wanted to remember often come to us in dreams or when we first awaken. The invention of the sewing machine needle by Elias Howe through a dream is an example familiar to most people. What are some examples from your own life? Rahima once had a dream that she was sent upstairs to see "Bernard." He was a kindly, gray-haired man, dressed in a business suit. When she told him what distress she was in and what a terrible time she was having, he said everything would soon change. He had her kneel down and touched her spine in various places, saying he was removing karma. She woke up higher than a kite, and with energy streaming through her. She later wondered if it had been St. Bernard she visited.

Prayer

Before, after, or instead of doing any of the suggestions in this chapter, try prayer if it is meaningful for you (perhaps even if it isn't). Ask that you experience forgiveness. Ask to be forgiven. Ask for healing. Ask for strength and for the ability to open. One of the birthing songs that has come through a friend in Colorado states:

I am opening up in sweet surrender to the
luminous lovelight of the Lord.
I am opening up in sweet surrender to the
luminous lovelight of the Lord.
I am opening. I am opening. I am opening.
I am opening.

Such a song can be sung like a mantra at a birth or a Blessing Way during pregnancy (Blessing Ways will be discussed in the next chaper). It is said that all real prayer is answered—we just don't know when.

Group Work

Part of the effectiveness of group work is the clear demonstration that we are not alone, that other women share our problems. Seeing the commonality of problems and the patterns that emerge help people to realize that they are in good company. The realization that other people share the same feelings or concerns can help alleviate loneliness, guilt and the feeling that the problem is HUGE. This is the power of sisterhood, the recognition that women can share and know other women's experiences just by having womanhood in common.

Group work with a therapist can be very rewarding, but so can group interactions with a childbirth educator who uses these or other exercises in helping couples explore the psychological aspects of birthing. Over the past decade many childbirth educators stopped trying to create conditioned responses in favor of helping women find the confidence and tools to cope with labor and delivery. The appearance of many thorough books on birth has also lessened the need to cover in class all the details of labor, delivery and postpartum; couples can go home and read the assigned chapter between classes. Time in class has thus been freed to focus on what couples haven't been able to do at home—emotional and group work.

Many of the exercises in this book were developed by the authors for their childbirth preparation classes. By sharing together, men and women are able to see the commonality of their experiences and to express things that might otherwise be left unsaid.

In addition to childbirth education classes, many childbirth organizations offer group support for women who have had a cesarean or parents who have lost a baby. Some of the national offices are listed in appendix of this book. Ask your local childbirth education groups or La Leche League leaders what exists in your community.

Informal groups can also offer a tremendous amount of support and healing. As midwives in Colorado, seven of us met regularly to study, discuss births and (once a month) to sweat together in an American Indian sweat lodge one of the women had built. Part of the sharing involved offering our impurities into the fire and sharing in prayer and words what we were wrestling with, feeling and wanting help with in our lives. Women sharing together create a tremendous power for healing.

A woman who will birth vaginally after a cesarean can find a great deal of support from a group of women who affirm her ability to give birth. One woman we know organized all her friends into a support group to help her stay encouraged and thinking positively during a difficult pregnancy with bleeding. Despite two previous cesareans (one of which had been a stillbirth), and a septate (divided) uterus, she went to full term and delivered the baby vaginally. She was tremendously grateful for all the support she received and felt it made a real difference.

A grieving circle is another activity a group of women can share with great benefit. We were first introduced to this practice by midwife/author Jeannine Parvati, who led a circle of women in sharing experiences related to loss in childbirth—stillbirths, abortions, miscarriages, or deaths of their own or other's babies. To do a grieving circle, everyone sits in a circle and it is explained that any person may start and tell her story of childbirth loss. Everyone is to listen without question or comment. When she is finished, the person on her left may either say ''I pass'' or may tell her story. Everyone continues around the circle until the first person is reached again. Then there can either be singing and prayer to end it, or you go around the circle again and tell the stories from an entirely different viewpoint, in an entirely different way. Grieving circles are very powerful in reminding us of the human condition and women's special connection to the powers of life and death.

Dealing with Emotions
Loss and Grief

A great deal has been written recently on loss and grief, starting with Kübler-Ross's work *On Death and Dying* and going through many books relating specifically to childbirth.[6] The one we recommend most highly is *Ended Beginnings* for anyone who has experienced childbirth-related losses.[7] If we include all of the loss of dreams through traumatic births, plus the birth of babies with defects, and the fact that more than one in three of the babies conceived in this country does not survive due to abortion, miscarriage or stillbirth, then the sisterhood of sorrow is large indeed.

Pregnant women are often reluctant to look at the possibility of childbirth loss, but understanding that grieving has its own cycle and that there is support available has proven invaluable for those who have had to go through such a tragedy. Certainly releasing past pain and loss is helpful in a present pregnancy.

Grief can be our reaction to any perceived loss, not only death. There can be a tremendous sense of loss about an ended relationship, an unexpected cesarean section, the birth of a child with a cleft lip, the birth of a boy when a girl was wanted (or vice versa). The most healing thing is to acknowledge these feelings in ourselves and in our friends without thinking, "I shouldn't be so upset." We cannot judge the scope of another person's pain, and grieving for a six-week fetus that has been lost can be as intense as grieving for a long-time friend or relative. Remarks such as, "At least you and the baby are both healthy" serve only to deny the emotions a person is feeling rather than to help her move through them.

Friends may feel uncomfortable after a family has lost a baby, and may avoid contact for fear of making the parents feel bad if they talk about the loss or seeming superficial and trivial if they talk about anything else. The most helpful thing to do is acknowledge the event and its pain and express your sympathy for the parents and then be available for whatever the parents want to do—talk about the loss or have a conversation about something else.

Couples who lose a baby through a miscarriage or stillbirth should know that actually seeing and touching the baby and saying goodbye can help in the healing process, but such contact should not be forced. Many hospital personnel are aware of the work of Klaus and others on newborn loss, and try to let the parents have time with their child; other hospitals still try to whisk the child away and "spare the parents the pain." But even a child with a birth defect rarely looks as bad as imagination paints it, and actually holding the baby who was present for such a short time can help the grieving. Naming the child and requesting the body for a simple funeral also helps some to live through the event. The parent's wishes should be respected; there's no "right" way.

Elisabeth Kubler-Ross was among the first to identify the stages of grief.[8] She went on to remind people that the stages must not be interpreted mechanically, for they interpenetrate one another. The important thing is that no feelings be invalidated or minimized by medical attendants or a well-meaning family. Over time there is a progression of emotions until the experience is worked through and acceptance is reached, and one can again look forward hopefully. Yet even when acceptance has occurred, it does not mean that you will not grieve on the baby's birthday or feel moments of anger or depression. But emotions have remained fluid, and a working-through process has occurred, preventing you from becoming stuck at any one of the phases. For example, a friend shared that she never saw her stillborn baby, and for many years after the birth she jumped every time the phone rang, in the irrational hope that it was the hospital calling to say there had been some mixup. Being able to see and hold the baby helps to work through that phase of denial.

Stages of grieving can be useful if you keep in mind the fluidity of emotions and don't use them as a recipe for "how to grieve":

● *Denial:* It is hard to accept that it really happened. Shock. It can't be true. It's a mistake.
● *Anger:* Fixing blame, usually on the people who cared for you most. Anger involves seeking an external reason for the happening. Whether or not it seems justified, allow yourself to feel this anger and see what comes next.
● *Guilt or Bargaining:* Suddenly you remember or seek for possible things you did that could have resulted in this inexplicable event. "I should have

taken more vitamins . . . We shouldn't have had intercourse . . . God is punishing me . . . If only I hadn't . . ."
● *Depression:* Fatigue can heighten the feeling of powerlessness and despair. Be sure to eat well, rest, and remember the hormonal changes that you are dealing with postpartum in addition to your grief.
● *Acceptance:* Growth and transformation; some kind of coming to terms with fate, God, the event; a gradual healing of the emptiness you have felt.

As a beginning midwife, Rahima was terrified of the prospect of delivering a baby who died in birth. She found it helpful to understand that grief has a cycle instead of being an endless emotional sea of turmoil. And she learned that everyone involved in a birth/death (attendants as well as parents) goes through his or her own grieving process, denial, self-questioning, anger, and so forth. Understanding this helped her feel that she would be able to go through such an experience rather than totally "freaking out" if and when it happened. This feeling helped her not only with all the births that were fine, but also when such a death did occur.

Each of us has experienced loss—either the loss of affection of someone we have loved, or the death of a parent, other relative, close friend or baby. In our own grief it is important to find the kind of support that we and other members of our family need. Children especially need to know they are loved and to understand that any negative thoughts they had did not kill the baby. They need to be reassured that everything is all right and that their parents will be all right. Men can also be deeply affected by the death of a baby with very few avenues of expression for their emotions. A great deal of "allowing" is needed during this time, so that couples can come through the experience together rather than feeling that the other partner is taking it too hard or not hard enough. Communication with each other and often with friends or counselors is essential for the grieving couple. One cannot predict in advance how a person will show grief. Accepting people for who they are and finding and giving support when one is hurting inside is not easy. But it is important to maintain trust and communication so that eventually you will be a couple who has had four children, one of whom died at eight-month's gestation; or a couple who had a certain experience with their first birth; or a couple who . . . . Reaching out to each other, holding hands even if you feel you are sinking, can help you re-emerge together rather than ending up cut off from each other.

Attention must also be put on physical healing.

Following a childbirth loss, a woman's hormones may change more rapidly than usual. And a cesarean delivery means recovering from major abdominal surgery as well as taking care of a new baby or mourning loss. The stress of loss and grief puts men and women at risk for other physical disorders and illnesses. Attention must be paid to sleep, nutrition, supplements and physical healing while emotions are so powerful.

Not only the death of a child causes grieving, but the birth of a child with a handicap also involves loss, with the added stress of coping with immediate medical concerns as well as adjustments that might be necessary throughout the child's life. Giving up a child for adoption can also involve grieving and loss. If this happened in your life, we recommend *To Love and Let Go* by Susanne Arms.[9]

Writing your experience, going through it with a friend who is the witness, visualizing your child and saying all the things you never could—all aid the healing process. It takes time, and there are few shortcuts. Acknowledging that it is all right to be feeling what you feel, that you are not going crazy or "taking it too hard," is the first step. Talking, writing, pondering can all help. Ritual and ceremony— either some you make up or those of your religion—can help bring a community together to share the grieving process. Support can also come through groups that are organized to help grieving parents. (See Appendix for national addresses of C/SEC, CPM, bereaved parents' groups and so forth; check with your local childbirth educators and La Leche League leaders to see what is available in your community.)

In the case of a premature or sick baby, there is often a double bind of not wanting to get too involved or too attached in case the baby doesn't make it. But the process of bonding and of "being there" for that small person can tip the scales and help dramatically in the baby's recovery. And the involvement will have been worth it regardless of the outcome. If the baby lives, you will be deeply concerned and involved, able to give the kind of parenting such a baby needs, much more easily than if you have maintained your distance while your baby was in intensive care. In fact, Klaus and Kennel's original studies on bonding were in the area of newborn loss and the effects of lack of bonding in the case of premature infants.[10] Their work showed the importance of the parents' being allowed to stay with their baby as much as possible in intensive care, touch even through the isolette, and breastfeed or express breastmilk for the baby. *Jonah Has a Rainbow* captures on film two parents' involvement with their baby from his birth at 6½ months of gestation through the celebration of his second birthday as the film closes.[11] Even if the baby dies, the heart will be larger for having loved. It is worth the risk!

Actually, grieving is universal in childbirth. There is *some* loss even with the birth of a healthy, longed-for child. There is the loss of the pregnancy, the loss of the two-ness of a couple with the birth of the first child, the loss of life as it used to be. An assimilation process must go on that involves letting go of the old and coming to terms with the new. Some women go through this process relatively easily; others blame their emotional instability on hormones; and some women find they are experiencing serious depression instead of ''baby blues.'' We will deal with postpartum grieving in Chapter 11; suffice it to say here that it is a normal part of the change and maturation each baby brings to its mother.

Anger

Anger is an emotion through which it is really easy to see the principle of ''banking,'' or saving up similar emotions. It's as if we save up all our annoyances until we have enough to ''cash in'' and really explode, often out of all proportion to the situation at hand. Panuthos uses the wonderful analogy of saving trading stamps: We save up each hurt, annoyance or loss until we fill the page, and then we feel justified in letting the emotions pour out of us.[12]

Anger can be very powerful, and may overcome rationality and the love that still exists between people. To work with present-time anger, it is best to start by letting off some of the steam through some extreme physical activity, like running, shouting, pounding pillows—or cleaning the entire house in twenty minutes. Assuming that we do not wish to frighten, threaten, or hurt the one with whom we are angry, this release allows us to express the physical rush or anger without necessarily unleashing it at him.

Once the fight-or-flight energy has been released, we are ready to:

1. Say we are angry.
2. Tell why we are angry.
3. Explain possible changes to prevent future disputes around the same topic (including changes in our own minds and habits).

When one is angry at a baby (or a corporation or bureaucracy), it is difficult to get satisfaction regard-ing behavioral changes, but be sure to let off the steam and state your anger in some way. Write it or paint it or dance it or organize a boycott, petition, or protest. Be sure the anger is not repressed and later taken out on someone else—or on yourself.

Do you have good habits in dealing with your anger? Many of us learned poor habits as children, because children are so often in no-power or manipulative positions when they become angry. Such situations teach repression or grudges or misplacement of anger. Some of us had parents or others around us who expressed their anger in nonproductive, violent ways, which we might now either duplicate or try to avoid by repressing our anger totally. Becoming aware of our anger patterns is especially important in parenting.

Tell here about any anger you have related to being pregnant, being in labor, being a mother.

_____

_____

_____

_____

Remember three recent times when you were angry and then analyze them according to the following questions (and others you may find appropriate):

1. **Describe or visualize the scenario—where, when, who was present, what was happening?**

_____

_____

_____

2. **What happened that led to your getting angry?**

_____

_____

_____

3. **Imagine some other possible feelings you could have had in that situation (e.g. humor, understanding, helpfulness, responsibility). Could any of these responses be appropriate for future situations?**

_____

_____

_____

4. **What did you do to express or not express your anger?**

_____

_____

_____

5. **Would you like to have acted differently? If so, what would you do differently?**

_____

_____

_____

6. **Would you consider the situation one where you could change the environment, adapt yourself, both, or neither?**

_____

_____

_____

Rage reduction is important if you want to create a harmonious birthing situation rather than approaching the medical community with so much anger from a previous birth that you're unable to get people to cooperate with you. Going into labor is not the time to go into battle! If you feel a lot of anger about a past birthing situation, try to work on it with a friend or counselor. Punching pillows is only more beneficial than chopping wood if it leads to insight and release of the causes behind the emotion rather than a simple letting off of steam.

After doing the letter writing exercise and/or really feeling your anger, try role-playing the situation. Take your "adversary's" part and try to feel what they were experiencing, what motivated them, how and why they did what they did. What did this experience show you?

_____

_____

_____

Most women are afraid of their anger. They are taught that it is an inappropriate emotion for a woman to feel. On the contrary, anger is a warning signal to us that something is wrong and that we need to affect change on some level. Often anger flares up when what we are really feeling is hurt or discounted by others. Expressing the underlying emotion rather than lashing out in anger will more often get what you really want.

Anger can have a very positive effect for social change. The fire of _Immaculate Deception_[13] and _Silent Knife: Cesarean Prevention and Vaginal Birth After Cesarean_[14] has changed childbirth for thousands of women in this country. But the delivery room is not the place to fight your battles. Fight them in the privacy of your own inner work, and then develop an effective strategy to achieve the kind of birthing you want, surrounded by supportive attendants with whom you can communicate and who trust your ability to give birth.

◆　◆　◆

SAVE THE CHILDREN

"Twenty-eight human beings, twenty-one of them children, die as a consequence of hunger every minute. This is equivalent to a Hiroshima every three days."

_my womb is the size of my fist
　is the size of my heart.
my womb could expand with a child
　if an egg were incited.
they say there are too many children
　and that's why they're starving
　　too weak for crying._

"No one dies of hunger because there is not enough to go around."

> *my womb is the size of my fist*
> *is the size of my heart.*
> *my fist becomes pregnant with anger*
> *and ripe for a revolution*
> *when I know that it's greed that leaves*
> *people hungry, people dying.*

"For less than the world spends on armies and weapons in one year we can eliminate hunger from our planet forever."

> *my womb is the size of my fist*
> *is the size of my heart.*
> *and my heart grows to bursting with caring*
> *that children are sick*
> *because rich men are not sharing.*

Terra

(Quotes from Hunger Project literature)

Depression

Depression is a gradual sinking, a heaviness of the heart due to restrictions of energy. It can be a necessary inward stage in the healing process of grieving in which case it can be immobilizing and very difficult to move through. But in its milder forms it is sometimes a way to avoid hurt or anger or facing a problem. Some people utilize depression as a manipulative way to gain attention, having probably learned it in childhood and activated it unconsciously. Here are some signs of depression:

Loss of appetite or over-
eating
Slouching posture
Avoiding people and fun
Not taking care of
yourself
Disinterest in life
Feeling of powerlessness
Sleepiness and/or
insomnia
Mumbling, low-powered
voice

Your own signs of depression:

_____

_____

_____

_____

These signs do not necessarily mean you are depressed, but if you notice that you are acting this way you may want to ask why. When you recognize depression in yourself during pregnancy, there is a need to open up and let the energy flow again. This can be accomplished in many ways. Here are a few suggestions, but create your own methods that best suit you. One key to breaking through depression during pregnancy or after the baby is born is to use love to get the energy flowing in a positive direction.

● Allow yourself to really cry or really get angry—sometimes calm can follow the storm.

● Do some physical movement—run, swim, do sit-ups, jump rope.

● Visit a favorite, jovial friend.

● Unselfishly do a good turn for someone.

● Make some clothes or a toy for your coming baby.

● Write a poem.

● Go to a party (and don't sit in the corner, moping).

● Visualize your body. See the energy in it. See the energy flowing more and more smoothly, nourishing you and your baby and flowing outwards, as well, to all those you love.

● Know what special songs inspire you and have them on hand to play or learn them to sing for the times you need an extra lift.

● If depression becomes a habit or is especially distressing, seek help in overcoming it from a friend, your spiritual advisor, or a professional counselor.

SELF RENEWAL

> *When I feel a prickly husk formed around me*
> *(or a shiny smooth one) I bury myself,*
> *nestle myself in the crack between sidewalks,*
> *or fly on vegetable wings*
> *away to an open space—*
> *there I plant myself in the soil,*
> *secret place where my covering can be safely*
> *burst.*

> *The sun gives freely, the sun gives . . .*
> *I grow—*
> *And grow—*
> *I'm roots and stem and leaves,*
> *sweet flowers and fruit,*
> *sweet mother again.*

Terra

Letting Go of Guilt

At this point perhaps we can recognize that feelings of guilt are a common part of the grieving process. If we are dissatisfied with our last birth experience, we can deny our feelings, or blame the doctors or our husband, or blame ourselves. One kind of feeling is not better or worse than another.

Just as we need to forgive others and recognize our own responsibility to move through anger, so we need to forgive ourselves and resolve to do better in the future to move out of feeling guilty. The nonproductive function of guilt is wallowing in self-blame to the point of becoming immobilized. It is natural to seek a cause. But knowledge and the facts may leave you not to blame—sometimes a cause simply is not known. But many women punish themselves by turning the blame inward and feeling as if they have failed or are worthless.

Guilt involves a dissatisfaction with ourselves, a feeling that we should have done differently. But usually we do the very best we can; it's just that sometimes we don't have all the information or we are keeping away the knowledge of consequences that on some level we must know. Whether ignorance, lack of responsibility or weakness resulted in our doing things during birth that we wish had gone differently, the important thing is to accept ourselves and to transform any feelings of guilt into the resolve to find out more and make different decisions in the future. Just coming to that point reflects inner growth and heightened awareness.

As women, we tend to blame and punish ourselves out of guilt, and that needs to stop. For example, if a woman is feeling bad about a cesarean birth and possible effects it has had on her baby, she needs to recognize that she did her best under those circumstances and made the best decisions she could at the time. She is not weak or a coward for having a cesarean; in fact, her physical pain postpartum was probably far greater than finishing labor would have been. She made a decision based on all of the facts available at that time, and one which put her baby's safety ahead of her own. If she is satisfied, there is no problem, for there is no right way to give birth. But is she is dissatisfied and feels that next time it must go differently, then she will take care of herself differently during this pregnancy, choose different attendants, and come to different attitudes and decisions about birthing that will help to shape and determine her next birth.

Guilt does not have to stay with us any longer than any other emotion. The introspective aspect of looking at our own weakness and complicity in an event can be valuable if it is used productively. The way guilt can be released is by accepting yourself for who you are (or were) and resolving to act on what you have seen and learned.

Further Words on Clearing Cesarean Births

When a woman has had a cesarean operation and develops a strong conviction that she wants a vaginal birth with her next child, she may find support for her decision is not readily forthcoming. America is one of the last remaining countries to give us the dictum, "Once a cesarean, always a cesarean." VBAC is much more accepted in other countries, but here finding a doctor or midwife who is really supportive can be a trying task. The greatest source of support is from other VBAC mothers, so we recommend you contact the Cesarean Prevention Movement and read *Silent Knife: Cesarean Prevention and Vaginal Birth After Cesarean.*[15]

Relatives are sometimes unsupportive, and even husbands sometimes don't understand the fervency of a woman's desire to birth vaginally. This calls for communication and acceptance of one another if true support is to arise without resentment. One woman wrote to us:

He acquired a stubborness and bitter attitude towards my quest for a vaginal birth after cesarean . . . . As I gradually changed my thinking on birth, he hung onto his. He bowed to the medical profession and believed they knew best and that I shouldn't question it. There were very few things about birth we agreed on and I cried a river, it seemed. So it was a very depressing situation and, as I mentioned before, I wanted to run away and give birth alone. I thank God for helping me through it all, granting me the privilege of vaginal birth and, too, for a strong marriage that held firm. Ironically, Jim was the one who, of his own will, immediately telephoned our childbirth educator with all the good news after we arrived home with the baby . . .

Once you have worked on releasing the events and emotions surrounding your cesarean birth, you need to work toward restoring your self-confidence and faith in normal birth. Choose from among the techniques we have suggested or use visualizations suggested in *Transformation through Birth*[16] or *Birthing Normally*.[17]

At a workshop sponsored by the Cesarean Prevention Movement where Nancy Cohen and Rahima were both speakers, cesarean couples wrote the following dialogues with Birthing Energy about their past experiences and their plans for upcoming vaginal births.

Me: (Woman): How do I keep you going?
B.E.: Focus on energy, don't think of outside forces.
Me: How do I learn to not hold it back?
B.E.: Think of the outcome—the baby.
Me: How do I keep others from slowing it down?
B.E.: Plan on educating them. You have to do it—no one else will. Get a midwife for a coach if you can't convince them.
Me: How will I remember everything?
B.E.: Practice until it is ingrained. Go through the process every day. Meditate on it. Read.
Me: Can I depend on it to carry me through?
B.E.: No. You have to work with it.
Me: Why did it stop in the second stage?
B.E.: Fear. You stopped working. You thought about the pain then. Before that you didn't think about it.
Me: What could I have done?
B.E.: Walked, moved.

Me: (Man): Can we really do it?
B.E.: All women's bodies are designed for it.
Me: I have read and prepared myself for this yet I am still really concerned.
B.E.: Great. Now show her you love her and that you are completely with her and there to help her And everything will be just fine.
Me: I know this VBAC is the most important thing in my wife's life right now and that she is completely sure she will do it. I ask for the same assurance.
B.E.: When the time comes you both will be together and work together. You will become one for the same end, a new human life which God gave all women the capability to do.

Me:(Midwife): Can we do it?
B.E.: Yes, you can. You're a capable, strong woman. Walk around, squat. Husband and I breathing together, feel the love and support. Relax.
Me: I love this baby. This is so right. Thank you God for seeing me through this beautiful birth. I waited so long for this. My husband is such a great support.
B.E.: You're great, you're doing fine.
Me: I feel I can't take much more.
B.E.: Yes, you can, you're terrific. You're doing well . . . You did it!

Me: (Man): What are you here for?
B.E.: I'm here to help you both.
Me: We don't need help. We took our class in Lamaze.
B.E.: You don't understand. I can help you. I'll be here when you need me.
Me: How can you help us?
B.E.: By showing you how to take advantage of the natural energy that the birth experience generates.
Me: Specifically, how?
B.E.: Touch her. Let her know how you feel; how she is doing; how much you love her. Tell her what this birth experience means to you. Relax. Be yourselves.

Me: (Woman): I welcome the contractions.
B.E.: This is my birth and it will not be like others and will take time.
Me: I feel the love of the attendants: the nurses, Patty and especially John.
B.E.: It will take everything you've got to do this, and that's why it's so special.
Me: I can't get a "Fifth Wind" and am so anxious to see this baby.
B.E.: Do you have the past behind you? Did you learn and grow from the first experience?
Me: We are stronger; I understand myself more deeply and can see that the experience gave me something special.

Me: (Woman): You're so scary.
B.E.: Why?
Me: I'm afraid of your taking over.
B.E.: I will, you know.
Me: I don't have to let you.
B.E.: I know.

Me: I want to let go.

B.E.: I know.

Me: I'm scared.

B.E.: You need me.

Me: I will go halfway with you.

B.E.: That won't work.

Me: I know. How do I let go?

B.E.: Accept yourself.

Me: But I don't like me. Nobody likes you
      unless you are important or give them
      something. I have nothing to give. Only
      small bits of me, and when I give it I get
      raped. If I give more I will be taken—
      possessed.

B.E.: I will not take from you. In accepting me
      you will become more.

Me: But there are strings attached.

B.E.: There are no strings.

Me: There is pain, expectations.

B.E.: There's pain anyway, and your
      expectations of yourself are greater.

Me: If I become one with you and don't
      live up to your expectations, you will
      leave and I will become empty.

B.E.: You are empty now.

Me: You are right.
      God, Energy of Creation
      energy of life
      source of joy
      beginner and ender
      giver and taker
      embracer
      giver of change
      every person
      one identity
      energy of existence
      outside of You
      there is emptiness.
      I embrace You
      and I become me.

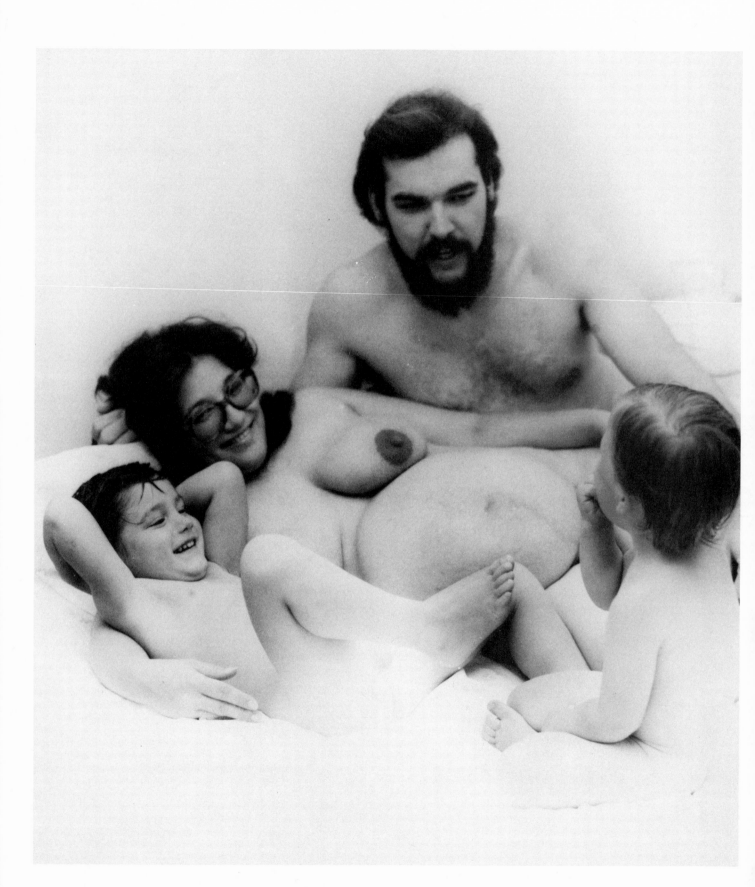

7
Fulfilling
Relationships

Pregnancy heightens a woman's sense of relationship, for she is never alone. The umbilical cord is a physical manifestation of the connectedness of mother and baby. As a pregnant woman, your life is being irrevocably changed during the journey to first-time mother or to mother-of-one-more-child. Relationship is being demanded of you, which is preparation for the task of mothering, when one must always be aware of the child's whereabouts and safety.

The demand to nurture, from one's physical substance during pregnancy, and from one's psychic or life-sustaining forces with a child, becomes an ongoing part of life. A tremendous growth in maturity and change of being are demanded of a new mother. The reward comes in giving birth and fostering new life, in your baby's smiles, in the positive changes you notice in yourself. The strength to go through these changes comes from within, from without, and from increased inner work. It isn't always easy, but growth seems always to win our consent sooner or later.

Pregnancy also brings you into increased awareness of your body and emotions, your needs and desires, your strengths and weaknesses, and your relationships with your partner, your other children, your own parents, and your spiritual wellspring. As we begin this chapter on ways of enhancing your relationships during pregnancy, spend a few moments taking stock of your current relationships.

How do you feel physically? Awful/Could be better/ Satisfied/Wonderful. Anything you could do to feel better?

_____

_____

_____

How is your relationship with your partner? Awful/Could be better/Satisfied/Wonderful. What things do you wish were different?

_____

_____

_____

How is your sexual relationship these days? If you're not satisfied, what would you like instead?

_____

_____

_____

How is your relationship with the baby? What primary emotions do you feel about him or her? Are there any ways you could be more in touch or any things you would like to do?

_____

_____

_____

How is your relationship with your other children, if applicable? If less than satisfying, what could you do to improve it? How are your relationships with friends? How is your relationship with your parents?

_____

_____

_____

_____

How is your relationship with God or your religious practice? What would you like to see happen?

_____

_____

_____

Enhancing Your Relationship with Your Baby

What do you know about your baby already? Do you have any sense of your baby's presence as a person? If so, when did this awareness first start? Have you had any dreams or presentiments about the baby's character or name? Some women receive such messages in dreams or meditations, while other women find singularly little insight into this child within them.

What have you experienced physically about the baby? Is he or she so active you think you'll turn black-and-blue from the inside out? Are there any patterns to your baby's movements? Does your baby seem to respond to music, loud noises, sunlight, relaxation, lovemaking?

Does your baby seem particularly large or small? Do people comment that you're carrying high or low? Have you heard your baby's heartbeat? It is accessible with a fetoscope from the sixteenth week, and towards the end of pregnancy your partner can often hear the heartbeat through an empty toilet-paper roll. Have you felt the baby's head, back, limbs? Ask your birth attendant to help you and your husband feel your baby, or refer to the section on palpation in *Special Delivery*.

How do you refer to the baby? Do you have a nickname you call the baby now? Do you talk to your baby? Do you talk about the baby with your husband and other children? Do they communicate with the baby directly through words and touch?

Do you sing to your baby? Even if you feel you can't sing, your voice is soothing and becomes recognized by your baby. Perhaps you'll develop a special song that will become your baby's. You'll be amazed at the calming effect such a song can have on a newborn.

The presence of the baby feels much larger than its small body and often seems to envelope the mother, giving her a special glow. After you have achieved a relaxed and meditative state, (discussed later in this chapter), open yourself to the presence of your baby. After a time, visualize the baby as he or she floats within the waters, rocked by your breathing and heartbeats. Do this at various times in your pregnancy, writing your experiences in your journal.

You can also lie next to your partner, with both his and your hands on your belly. Try experiencing this baby/being. There are several guided visualizations which can help *both* parents to be more in touch with the baby on a tape called "The Child Within" by Leni Schwartz[1] or "Birthing Tools" by Laura Hersey.[2]

Enhancing Your Relationship with Your Body

Physical Changes/ Emotional Changes

Dealing with all of the visible and invisible changes in one's body, emotions, lifestyle and relationships brought about by a pregnancy and the birth of a baby can sometimes leave a woman feeling that she's adrift in a sea of change. Keeping one's emotional equilibrium can be helped by keeping perspective and by talking with your partner or friend. But the underlying physical component of the emotions of pregnancy should not be overlooked!

Many times a physical change can drastically change our emotional state. This is obvious in the case of a warm bath, a brisk walk, or going for a swim. More subtle but equally important are longer-range factors such as feeling like a "beached whale" or feeling run down all the time. Emotional equilibrium can be fostered by maintaining good physical habits (which are easier to list than they are to follow!):

1. Exercise and massage. Exercise can release tension, promote better blood circulation, build stamina and create more red blood cells to carry oxygen to both you and your baby. Water sports are especially recommended since they return you to a state of weightlessness and grace. Massage can help improve the circulation as well as release tension.

2. Rest. To sleep whenever you are tired sometimes seems impossible, but it is definitely a necessity for good health, especially during pregnancy, postpartum and breastfeeding. If, on the other hand, tiredness is a habit, check for anemia, increase your exercise, try changing daily routines to avoid boredom, or have a complete physical checkup.

Because most women are reacting against the image of pregnancy as an illness, they feel they have to keep holding their own and not appear weak. But the work of building a baby is very real and very demanding, and the Superwoman routine of working at a fulltime job until your due date can be both physically and emotionally draining. Setting the timer to rest fifteen minutes a day, as one woman did who was developing complications, does not show enough of a change in attitude toward oneself and one's body to do much good.

3. Good Nutrition. Good nutrition is hard to define, and is actually as individual and changeable as we ourselves. To have good nutrition, we must be sure to eat the necessary basics and then check ourselves out individually to see if there are any special needs still unfulfilled. It requires study about what each body needs to do its work correctly, and, sometimes, professional advice. Good eating and digesting can help us relax by keeping nerves in good order. Vitamin C, B-complex vitamins, and calcium especially help with relaxation.

Good chewing, calmness at mealtime, and avoidance of late-night meals help digestion and absorption of what we eat.

4. Personal Care. Sometimes better personal care can wash away tension and bad feelings. Washing before meals, before bed or after a trying experience can be a moment of bodily awareness and letting go. A shower can be as cleansing to the spirit as a good thunderstorm, and a warm bath is a well-know calmant.

Improving Nutrition

Improving your nutrition helps you feel better, and it is even more important for your baby. Results of nutritional studies show that mothers who get sufficient daily vitamins, minerals and protein during their pregnancy have fewer cases of metabolic toxemia of pregnancy, and fewer cases of premature, low-birth-weight and stillborn babies. The labors of such women are more often completely normal. After the birth, their babies have fewer cases of colds and hyperactivity. What we eat during pregnancy makes a *big* difference, immediately and later on.

What should you be eating? Individual needs vary according to metabolism and your own unique physical condition. But you need sufficient daily calories through wholesome foods from all of the food groups to enable your baby and the placenta to grow in the healthiest way. You also need sufficient salt and water in your diet and should *not* restrict these, even if you are experiencing swelling of the hands and ankles. Avoid calorie-reducing diets and diuretics, and if you are having any problems that cause your doctor concern, be sure to read *What Every Pregnant Woman Should Know: The Truth about Diet and Drugs in Pregnancy* by Gail and Tom Brewer.[3]

Eating 80 to 100 grams of high-quality protein a day serves to prevent toxemia. In fact, if you are showing protein in your urine, a sign of early toxemia, you need to *increase* your protein intake. (See Brewer's book or *Preventing Nutritional Complications of Pregnancy, A Manual for SPUN Counselors* published by the Society for the Protection of the Unborn through Nutrition and available through Informed Birth and Parenting, Box 3675, Ann Arbor, MI 48106.)

Here are suggestions for evaluating your nutrition, which can be implemented using Brewer's book or *Special Delivery:*

● **Write down everything you eat for three days. Figure the number of grams of protein using the tables in the above books. Are you within the 70 to 100 grams/day range? Only halfway?**

● **Think of something you often eat that is high in sugar or chemical additives. If you would like to cut it out of your diet, think of what qualities it has (sweet, crunchy, whatever), when you eat it (when bored, reading, upset), and think of a more nutritious food that would satisfy some of those same appetites. Stock the new item, and get rid of the old. Is there a "frontier area" of something in your personal or family's diet that you have been meaning to change (buying bottled water, eating less refined sugar, cutting down on fried foods, whatever)? List what it would take to do it, then do it (pick just one thing to start).**

● **Are there times when you go too long without eating, and reach for junk food because you're starving? Can you keep a nutritious snack for such emergencies in the car, at your job, or wherever you often get caught?**

Increasing Your Comfort During Pregnancy

Many of the discomforts associated with pregnancy seem to be helped by nutritional supplements. For example, taking calcium can help cramping of muscles in the calves or other parts of the body. Ginger is now becoming known as a help for morning sickness. (Most sources recommend 500-mg capsules of ginger taken three at a time during the day to stay ahead of feelings of nausea; it is also being used for nausea in motion sickness, an interesting parallel).[4]

Backache can be helped with physical exercises such as those taught in childbirth preparation classes or illustrated in *Special Delivery*. Massage and pressure point work can also alleviate many of the discomforts of pregnancy. One can never have too much massage. It is a natural adjunct to relaxation exercises or bedroom play with your partner. Exchange massages on alternate nights. If you have a professional massage, remember not to lie flat on your back on a hard table for a long period of time in your last months of pregnancy. Circulation may be decreased from the weight of the baby on your major veins and this can cause fetal distress. The side relaxation position is best in this case.

Where does it hurt? List any general or specific complaints you have been having, and list at least three things you could do or get someone else to do to help you feel better. You deserve it.

Increasing Relaxation

Relaxation is an important skill for everyone, but it is especially useful during pregnancy, birth and mothering. If you can develop a relaxation response to your partner's touch, he can be more effective at helping you to relax during labor; you are much more likely to be able to relax to his touch than to his simply telling you to relax your shoulders! You need to learn to use your mind to relax your body, because your body will tense involuntarily as a contraction begins. You then need to tell your body, "Thank you for the message, but this all right, and we're going to stay here and relax." Staying relaxed is the main key to preventing pain in labor. Your uterus naturally contracts and relaxes; but your muscles can stay tensed for hours, which is extremely painful as lactic acid builds up. Imagine how painful it would be to hold your biceps flexed for eleven hours (if you could do it!).

There are many techniques of relaxation, all of which are designed to help us remember the relaxed state, and to condition us to enter it more easily whenever we choose. People usually find some techniques more effective than others, so be sure to try several. However, do practice a method for a week before discarding it, as experience may improve its usefulness. Practicing relaxation regularly helps to keep tension from building up and allows you to reach deeper and deeper states of relaxation.

Techniques for Relaxation

For all techniques, find a time and place where you can relax. It should be quiet, warm, calm, solitary, with subdued lighting. Unplug the telephone. Put away thoughts that may run through your mind by letting them run their course—don't bother to argue, repress or confront them. Sit or lie comfortably with loosened clothing, bare feet, uncrossed legs and arms. Bedtime, or when first waking, is often the best opportunity for some quiet time.

Whole-Body Relaxation

With this technique, you get into a relaxed position with eyes closed and then relax each part of your body in an orderly manner, from toes to top of head. This is a helpful phrase to proceed with: "I am aware of my toes. I feel my toes becoming more and more relaxed." Replace "toes" with the next appropriate part, as you move throughout your body. Be sure to remember your back, your vagina and uterus and your other internal organs. At the end, feel your entire body totally relaxed. If tension remains in any spot, go there with your mind and help it relax further.

This technique is helpful in becoming aware of your whole body. It teaches you where you tend to be habitually tense. It also strengthens the suggestion in your mind that, whenever you desire, you can consciously relax any part of your body.

Relaxation Visualizations

The most effective relaxation visualizations are those that tune in to your personal memories and desires. They include not only seeing with your imagination, but also "hearing, smelling, tasting, and feeling." Try these examples and then go on to create your own. Practice makes this more effective. You may want to first try doing some whole-body relaxation, and then visualizing. This will link visualization even more strongly to the relaxed state. (Review the discussion of visualization in the last chapter.)

● Imagine yourself in your favorite peaceful room, meadow, at the beach, in bed.
● Imagine floating in warm water, or sinking into warm sand, lying under the hot sun.
● Imagine all tension being exhaled with each out-breath and relaxation being inhaled with each in-breath. Tension might look like a dirty, gray color, and relaxation, like a mellow green.
● Feel yourself melting into the floor or bed, getting heavier and heavier.
● Count backwards from ten to one and feel more and more relaxed with each number. You might visualize each numeral as you count.

Breathing Relaxation

Breathing is a natural relaxer. Take a deep breath and exhale. Feel how you automatically relax as you let your breath go. You can enhance this effect by consciously participating in it. Use the visualization for exhaling tension and inhaling relaxation. When you notice tension in a certain part of your body, breathe through it. For example, if your shoulder is tense, feel it expand with air as you inhale, as though it is inhaling also. Then feel it relax as you and your shoulder exhale.

One common form of meditation-relaxation is to lie or sit quietly and just be aware of your breathing. Don't force or control how you breathe, just watch it as it comes and goes, like the waves at the seashore.

Differential Relaxation

This form demonstrates the possibility of relaxing most of your body while your uterus is contracting during labor. With this technique, you get into a relaxed position (perhaps doing whole-body relaxation or visualization first), and then tense up one shoulder or your buttocks while keeping the rest of your body relaxed. You can combine it with touch relaxation by tensing just one set of muscles and then releasing to your partner's touch. This takes practice, so don't be discouraged the first time you try to do it.

A similar type of labor relaxation practice is to have your partner simulate a contraction by squeezing the inside of your thigh. This will not feel like a contraction, yet it can help you realize that by relaxing and using deep breathing, you *can* learn to let the pain be there without being overwhelmed by it.

Touch Relaxation

Touch relaxation uses your partner's help in a much more pleasant way. Your partner must learn to recognize when and where you are tense. You will tense some part of your body. When he sees that you are tense, for example, in your jaws, he will gently touch your jaws with his hands, drawing the tension gently from you, as though his hands were magnetized to attract it. You will release the area he touches, imagining the tension going into his hands, and feeling more relaxed afterwards.

Practicing touch relaxation is necessary to build tension release as an automatic response to being touched. Each partner needs to give feedback to the other, so that each can improve in technique. Switching roles gives each person perspective and a chance to relax.

Increasing Body Awareness

How you feel about yourself and your body affects your birthing as well as your sexual relationship with your partner. It is helpful to be able to experience your bodily nature and instincts to give birth in the easiest possible way. Animals need no childbirth classes or breathing techniques! The instinctive aspects of birthing can be encouraged by becoming more aware of your body.

● **Be alone and naked in front of a mirror (full length, if possible). Look at your body as it is. Listen to your mental and emotional reactions. Where do they originate? Try to let any negativity go and focus on positive, voluptuous qualities.**

● **Take a luxurious bath. Afterward, be alone and naked in a quiet, peaceful setting. Touch your body all over, and feel how it is changing. Dance with it, feeling your changing center of gravity.**

● **Photograph your body periodically throughout and after pregnancy and see how it changes.**

● **Name five adjectives describing your body before pregnancy.**

● **Name five adjectives describing your body now.**

● **Name your feelings about these changes.**

● **How does your partner react to these changes?**

● **In privacy, and when you have plenty of time, take a hand mirror and look at your genitals. If you get a plastic speculum (available at women's clinics or birthing supply companies), a mirror and a flashlight you can even look at your cervix! (Talk to your midwife or doctor about this and they can give you more information.) If you learn to know and like your perineum through perineal massage, there will be less likelihood of perineal tears or need for an episiotomy. Do pelvic floor exercises (see the following pages for information on these techniques).**

• Look at some paintings and photos of pregnant women, fertility goddesses, and Rubenesque, voluptuous women to increase your appreciation of your own ripe body. This is to counteract the emphasis in our culture on the undernourished look.

• Practice listening to your body and it will be more of a friend. Eat when you feel hungry; learn to differentiate a nervous craving from a body hunger. Urinate and have bowel movements when you first notice you need to, instead of "holding" it. Sleep when you are sleepy. Stretch and relax when you feel tense.

• Have some massage sessions with your partner. Give each other feedback on how different techniques feel; you will both learn how to give great massages, as well as practice clear communications. By making massage separate from sexual relations, it can be more relaxed and purely sensual. This can also give you an alternate form of sensual sharing.

Becoming More Uninhibited

To complete a normal, unmedicated labor and birth successfully, it is helpful to let go and be at one with the force of the contractions, doing as they do. They might lead you at some point to sing or chant or moan or shake. Some women might find this kind of activity goes against their physical modesty or their desire to be self-controlled at all times.

Here are some suggested exercises in being uninhibited:

1. Take a movement class which lets you flow rather than be totally in control, such as belly dancing or dance improvisation (Clear this with your midwife or doctor, if you have any questions of safety.)

2. Start singing out loud: sing to your baby, sing to your partner, sing to yourself and to life.

3. When you have the urge, seduce your partner, perhaps at an unexpected time or place.

4. While making love, be noisier than you ever dared to be before.

5. Practice expressing yourself physically and verbally. In appropriate situations, use your hands and sound effects when you talk; let yourself yawn, burp and fart; grunt when you have to exert yourself; if you are all wound up and feel like screaming, do it; try being melodramatic sometimes.

Enhancing Your Relationship with Your Partner

Sexuality in Pregnancy

Pregnancy and birth, which are an intimate and integral part of a woman's and a couple's sexual life, naturally have an impact on your experience of sexuality and desire for lovemaking, not only during pregnancy, but also after the birth and for as long as you are nursing. In Chapter 2 we discussed women's varying sexual responses during pregnancy to reaffirm that no matter what is happening to you, you are in good company.

Keys to a couple's sexual relationship during pregnancy are how a woman feels physically, how she feels about herself, and the quality of sharing between the two people. Are you and your husband friends? Is the bedroom a welcome place for sharing physically the love that is between you, or is it an arena in which problems from the day, or from years of sexual nonencounter with one another, result in yet another standoff or loss of ground?

Sexuality is an important element of marriage. The fact that it is one of the areas of highest confusion in human relationships makes it more difficult to do work in this area. Suggestions we have made for clearing the past can be applied to the area of sexuality, but the muddle in which most couples find themselves requires a lot of forgiveness and clear consciousness to escape the labyrinth of emotions associated with as powerful and creative an act as sexual sharing. The creative energy of the universe that is felt as sexuality is, in its purest form, very spiritual and is the life force of the world. It is the energy some religions want to sublimate out of the body; others try to recognize its spiritual reality within and through the body.

Sexuality is something each person experiences, since each is a polarized part of the universe. It is not just something experienced *between* people. Both the universality and the individuality of women's experience of sex was given by Sheila Kitzinger in her book by that name.[5] As male and female, we participate in the sexuality of the world, and there is no scarcity of it. (You may doubt that statement if you remember times of being so exhausted that there wasn't any sexuality to be found, but it was there, and it always came back!).

On a night when you're not going to have intercourse, agree with one another to try feeling sexual energy. Touch, kiss, focus neither on one another nor on the space in between, just open to the infinite sexual energy that pulses through the world. Breathe deeply and in a relaxed way, all the way down into your sexual area; let your breath freely move and breathe with any waves of energy you may feel. Make contented noises or sighs when you feel something, so you can communicate that with your partner; you'll probably find you start feeling similar things. Move your body, especially your pelvis, with any waves of energy you may feel. The same kind of energy that can stream out of a woman's breasts can be channelled by a man through his hands. Have him put his hands on your lower belly as you both open to the flow of sexual energy. When you've played enough, kiss and go to sleep. If you didn't experience anything in response to that exercise, devise your own and try it another time. If you did experience any sexual flow, you may be asking, "What, no intercourse? Won't his balls turn blue and fall off? What about that wasted erection?" Truly, there is nothing harmful in a man's experiencing arousal or even intercourse without ejaculation. There are not only no negative physical effects, but men who practice this technique often find both increased sexuality and also new vitality in all areas of their lives. (See Jolan Chang's two books *The Tao of the Loving Couple* and *The Tao of Love and Sex*.[6])

The ability to let sexual energy come and go without its invariably leading to intercourse or ejaculation can be very freeing in a relationship. Many women feel less than satisfied when men ejaculate quickly once penetration occurs (Kinsey reported the average to be about three minutes!). They are also dismayed by how quickly men want to get to intercourse. Even the word *foreplay* places intercourse in a position of primary importance. Deciding to give up intercourse or ejaculation, even some of the time, is one way of getting around a sexual impasse. Whether a man comes to this experience through non-ejaculation or realizing that he can have several ejaculations without losing an erection is of secondary importance compared to the freedom that comes when sex is a true sharing rather than a way of "getting your rocks off." The quality of the energy shared may be much better than in usual encounters, which should be satisfying for both partners. And the quality of intercourse can improve too.

The tremendous power of creative sexual energy is especially available when a couple is open to the possibility of conceiving and nurturing a new life. Whether or not you experienced this quality of energy when you conceived your child, it is possible to open to it now and experience it during your pregnancy. It is not necessary to have a conscious conception to have a conscious pregnancy. It is sometimes possible to experience this energy when you are not pregnant, but then you had better be careful because you're probably fertile!

Try lying naked together when you are relaxed and have plenty of time, and have him put his hand on your belly. Feel the baby, feel your sexuality, feel the energy that is creating this child in your marriage. This involves a kind of opening to make contact with very powerful energy. One key to maintaining contact with this kind of energy during your pregnancy seems to be to maintain awareness of the baby during lovemaking. This makes it possible to tune into the higher energy of creation in a way which denying the presence of the baby precludes. But there are no guarantees—see what works for you.

Another key to nurturing lovemaking during pregnancy or at any other time is to communicate during and after intercourse and to stop if it doesn't feel good. This doesn't only mean stop if it hurts, but also if it is mediocre or if you are mentally or emotionally distracted, for whatever reason. It is amazing how much women suffer in silence rather than risk censure or hurting their lover's ego or wasting his erection. It is also amazing how oblivious men can be to their lover's emotional state. This, of course, compounds a woman's hurt and resentment, as she is hard pressed to understand how he can be having such a good time while being so out of touch with her.

Men and women tend to be very different in their experience of emotions and sexuality. Women tend to be much more at home in the emotional/intuitive realm and the realm of nurturing; men, tend to be simultaneously grounded in the physical and at home in abstract thought, while being weak in the middle sphere of emotion and nurturing. This is not a startling observation to anyone who has contemplated masculine and feminine, left and right brain, and so forth; and it does not say that men can't be nurturing or that women can't think. But it does offer clues as to why intercourse is so meaningful for a woman, and cannot generally be separated from her emotions, either those about events of the day or about her lover. This is not often the case for her mate, who can set aside other experiences or feelings in order to approach and enjoy the physical aspects of intercourse. His pleasure is not so interwoven with his feelings about his partner. This helps to explain how a man can be oblivious to his partner's feelings during intercourse, while it is impossible for her to ignore her feelings.

Another example of this difference in outlook is that a man can *think* that his marriage is basically fine (abstract thought about the spiritual connection) and spend his time working long hours to buy a new house (providing in the physical realm). Only when he sees his wife reading ''Single Apartments for Rent'' ads does he know there is anything wrong. That is an extreme case, but it actually happened to a man we know. Most men are slightly more in touch with their emotions than our friend, but being comfortable in the emotional sphere and trusting these emotions are things that men are only coming to through increased consciousness and inner work.

Natural differences between masculine and feminine, as well as differences in character, can help to create balance within a relationship to the benefit of both. But, while individuals can balance each other through complementary qualities, a lack of common meeting ground can also lead to misunderstandings. Clearly, working toward growth and balance within oneself can help each person be more complete and relationships be more balanced.

Women's consciousness-raising has helped many of us to understand our nature as women, but we still tend to understand men less well. Consciousness-raising in this area needs to happen, not only for men themselves, but also for women as we relate to our husbands and sons. For example,

understanding the male need to encounter resistance in physical matter can help us understand the play of boys (of all ages). Understanding the differences between the ordinary consciousness of men and women can help lessen the sense of blame and misunderstanding which often exists, especially in the area of sex. Open communication, respect, forgiveness, and the willingness to grow can take you in the right direction without any fancy explanations. (How's that for a woman's statement, completely illustrative of the above points?)

The following are some practical suggestions concerning sex during pregnancy.

● Unless advised otherwise by your health care provider, sexual intercourse is not harmful during pregnancy until the waters break during labor. If you have any doubts or questions about sex, be sure to discuss them with your partner and/or health care provider before they are magnified in your mind. For example, many women experience slight spotting around the time of one of their first few missed periods. This can be a normal function of hormonal changes early in pregnancy, but the spotting can become associated in your mind with intercourse the preceding night and lead to needless anxiety. Previous miscarriage is an area where you need to be clear as a couple about intercourse; intercourse may be perfectly fine, or it may be contraindicated, as in the case of repeated miscarriages. Check with your health care provider to get more facts if you have any anxieties in this area. Also check your own intuitive knowing.

● It is not dangerous or unusual to have contractions during or right after making love during the second half of pregnancy. You could think of them as hugging the baby. Arousal and nipple stimulation release natural oxytocin, which causes the uterus to contract during orgasm. It will encourage labor only if your body is ripe to go into labor anyway.

● Urinating after intercourse can help decrease the chance of bladder infections.

● The sexual desire of pregnant women may vary greatly from woman to woman and for any individual woman from trimester to trimester. Don't think there is any right or wrong way to feel.

● It is all right not to want sexual intercourse. But it needs to be worked out with one's partner in a conscious way to avoid causing problems.

● Positive sexual experiences are a way for you to tune in to each other as a couple. When there is a problem about sex that is kept secret, it builds barriers between you. Talk to your partner!

● It's not uncommon for a man to feel uncomfortable about making love at some point in pregnancy. He may think he'll hurt or upset the baby, or he may feel as if a third party is watching. He might find the changes in your body bewildering or even unattractive. Be sure to talk about these feelings together.

● If you are too tired to make love in the evening, try it in the morning, afternoon, or middle of the night. Try sharing energy instead of being orgasm-oriented.

● Be sure to try new positions to find what is most comfortable as the baby becomes more and more of a presence between you. Some possibilities include: woman on top, woman lying on her side with partner curled around her ("spooning"), woman on hands and knees or sitting on his lap (facing one another) while leaning back, supported by her hands.

● Do something fun—give yourselves an exotic evening. Appreciate that you don't yet have the baby waking up in the middle of lovemaking!

Problem-Solving in Relationships

Disagreements can arise at any time in a relationship, but during pregnancy there seem to be so many important issues to discuss. In addition to the usual problem of stretching the paychecks and child-rearing questions with other children, there are important issues about the place of birth, finding an attendant and circumcision, to name just a few. Your husband will need to inform himself on these issues just as you do, and you will need to share the information you are gaining with him.

In the next chapter we offer specific exercises for helping to clarify values, because understanding where the other person is coming from can help in finding the best solutions for the two of you. Any kind of difficulty becomes easier when put into perspective. All things, especially our minds, change if we wait for a little while. Here are some exercises to help with gaining perspectives on difficulties.

Time perspective

Get into a relaxed state by releasing tension from your body as you travel through it with your mind's eye. Try to see the problem. See what it was a week ago, a month ago. See what it might be a week from now, in six months, one year, five years from now. See a graph of your lifespan. See how much of the graph would relate to this problem in your life. See a graph of recorded history. See how much of it would relate to your life and problem.

Space perspective

Get into a relaxed state. See yourself with your problems. See yourself in your home. See yourself in your block or mail route. See yourself in your city, your county, your state, your country. See yourself and your problem from a space station, from the moon, from the sun, from another solar system. See yourself and your problem from another galaxy.

Attitude perspective I

Get into a relaxed state. You are now a movie director. Your problem is a situation that is being made into a movie. You've decided to make your dramatic situation into a comedy, maybe even a slapstick comedy. See what the movie would be like.

Attitude perspective II

Get into a relaxed state. Count your blessings. Compare your life with a pregnant woman in another country who lives on the streets and must beg for food.

Energy in Relationships

In our relationships we continually weave between being active and receptive, self-sufficient and dependent, giving and receiving. Certain patterns emerge over time, or within a given relationship. Do you know someone who brings out the worst in you? Whenever you are around them you feel totally incompetent and weak? Or is there someone who is always creating a problem from which you have to save them? Do you find that you are fiercely independent and would rather do everything yourself, or are you content to let everything drift along and it doesn't really matter that everything remains unfinished?

We relate to the energy of birth in much the way we relate to energy surrounding us in ordinary life. A woman does not become radically different in labor, doing things totally out of character. Indeed, giving birth is part of the continuum of life and is colored by all our attitudes and life patterns. Sometimes during labor and birth a woman's ordinary ways of relating to the world are played out with greater intensity, amplified by the power of the hormones and energy flowing through her. One friend was a dancer and had a dozen people at her birth—she needed that audience! Another was a single mother who felt she had to do everything herself. She arranged to do the LeBoyer bath herself, but said in retrospect that she was so shaky and everyone was so worried she would drop the baby, that she wasn't able to convey relaxation to her new daughter. She wished, in fact, that she had let someone else hold her in the water.

Activity and Passivity in Birth

One aspect of how we live our lives that can be important at the time of birth is how active or passive we usually are. Passivity/Activity has to do with how we adapt to the energy flow around us or how we adapt that energy flow to us. Passive behavior is that which totally "goes with the flow." Active behavior is that which changes the environment to suit what we have in mind. It is helpful during labor to be passive enough to allow the baby to come down and yet active enough to help push the baby out. Being flexible yet directed during pregnancy can help you stay that way during labor.

1. Name some of your recent active behaviors.

_____

_____

_____

2. Name some of your recent passive behaviors.

_____

_____

_____

3. Do you tend towards activity or passivity?

_____

_____

_____

It is helpful in birth to have the passive qualities of *trust in others* and in the Universe and the *humility* to accept what one is given, rather than forcing life always to fit one's own wishes. If you have the opportunity to try the following exercises, observe your reactions and any growth that occurs through them.

1. Allow your body to go totally limp. Let your partner move your body around, while you stay relaxed.

2. When you are with someone else and you are all deciding what to do for the evening (for example), let them decide and feel peaceful about it. You can try this with any decision that, after all, does not mean very much.

3. Practice being a servant to someone you trust. Devotedly do as they ask.

4. Play music on the radio or stereo and dance to it, allowing your body to move as it wishes to the music.

It is also valuable in birthing to have the active qualities of *trust in yourself* and *assertiveness* in expressing what you think and feel. Validate your own active behavior by assessing the following:

1. Write down all of the creative things that you have done in the last week (not just artistically creative—include innovations in your everyday life).

_____

_____

_____

_____

2. Write down some new creative experiences you'd like to have. Cross them off the list after you do them.

_____

_____

_____

_____

_____

_____

3. Start a new project you've been dreaming about, or complete one that's been on the back burner.

4. Be the dominant, active partner next time you make love.

5. Sing, make music, play in sports, dance, instead of being passively entertained.

Interdependence in Birth

Dependence/Independence has to do with being able to accept help and support from others and being able to be self-supporting. Unduly dependent behavior is that which seeks a lot of help and energy from others. Examples are: letting others make decisions; expecting others to know and provide what you want or need (even when you don't tell them). Independent behavior works towards being self-supporting, and in pregnancy involves informing oneself and taking responsibility for decisions. Yet independence can also be carried too far, so that you are bearing all the burden yourself without allowing the help and sharing that your mate, friends and attendants can provide. During labor, it is important to be able to accept help when it is needed, yet be able to feel self-confident enough to give birth to the baby.

Assessing Your Ability to Accept Help (examples)

1. Use affirmations, such as: "I can accept help without losing my own power." What reactions do you have?

_____

_____

_____

_____

2. Ask help in doing something; practice feeling OK about it.

3. Become aware of when you are not feeling OK about accepting help from others. Name some instances and your feelings about the situation; list some alternative reactions.

_____

_____

_____

_____

_____

_____

_____

4. If you find it difficult to accept help from others, why do you believe you are that way? Is it always a functional way to behave? What need in you does it fulfill to be totally independent?

_____

_____

_____

_____

_____

Assessing Your Independence (examples)

1. Use affirmations, such as: "I can accomplish this (name the specific behavior) through my own strength." What reactions do you have?

_____

_____

_____

2. Rather than ask help to accomplish a task, try to do it all on your own, even if it takes longer to learn how to do it. Start out with small, simple tasks and work your way up to doing something all by yourself that you never would have imagined that you could do independently.

3. Become aware of when you are acting dependent. Identify some instances and write how you felt inside. Next to them, suggest some more independent reactions and behaviors.

_____

_____

_____

_____

_____

4. If you have difficulties being independent, why do you believe you act that way? What need in you does it fulfill? How could you fulfill it differently?

_____

_____

_____

_____

Developing Acceptance

Although it is possible for us to influence our physical health (and what happens to us) by our confusion or clarity, it is not always possible to have everything the way we want it! Because of our limited vision on this level, we are not always able to see why something we don't like occurs or the possible beneficial effects that it may have. This is true in our lives and is even more true when we include the lives and destinies of others. For example, we may do everything "right" and still have a child who is born with special needs. As new parents we can only work toward acceptance and trying to help that child realize his or her own potential to the fullest.

Or it sometimes happens that a baby goes into distress during labor or that some other complication totally changes the course of what we had anticipated. Sometimes a mother attempting a VBAC still requires a cesarean for her second baby. This doesn't mean that we shouldn't work with our emotions and intentions and try to be as clear as we can, but there are no guarantees. Sometimes we don't like the lessons we need to learn, or find it hard to see the good hidden in them. One value is the growth that can often be involved in coming to accept what we don't understand. Often forgiveness of oneself, of others and of God are issues that get resolved. Patience is also a component of acceptance, which is important during pregnancy, labor and childcare. It is helpful in living with the inconveniences and discomforts of pregnancy, and can be especially useful in your ninth month. Only 5 percent of all babies are born on the due date, so relaxing and letting nature take its course are clearly recommended. Patience is often required in labor as well, when you need to stay in the present moment instead of railing about how long it is taking.

Less Tangible Relationships

Trusting in the will of God, the creative power of the universe, or the wisdom of nature (whatever words you want to call it) can be important during pregnancy. We have to do our share through being informed, eating well, having prenatal care and making arrangements for the birth, but we also have to affirm our trust in the process of birth and acknowledge that life and death are questions not wholly in human control. The Sufis say, "Tether your camel, then trust in God." You can neither let him run free and trust God to keep him there nor think that all the knots of your own device will prevent his getting lost or stolen if God wills it.

Think about your own attitudes and beliefs about birth and the order of the universe. Share these thoughts with your partner.

Rudolf Steiner, founder of the path of spiritual development called anthroposophy and of the Waldorf schools, often recommended that a pregnant woman meditate daily on a picture of "The Sistine Madonna" by Raphael. Steiner saw in this picture a particularly clear representation of both the essence of motherhood and the development of the human ego. Steiner also felt that attention to art, beauty and music were especially beneficial for the pregnant mother and baby, but that she should avoid spiritual/physical exercises that engage the same life forces that are forming her child (eurythmy or breathing exercises for example).

The Value of Affirmations

Our values and beliefs influence what happens to us by aligning our energy with them and making it more likely that they will manifest in our lives. Much of our life has a self-fulfilling character. We seem to attract what we fear, or we can often say, "I knew that would happen to me."

Since what we say about ourselves (positive or negative) strongly influences what actually unfolds in our lives, it is possible to take advantage of this by creating or using positive affirmations. Repeating or writing affirmations such as the following can help you to realize their truth and to identify and release any blocks from the past that may stand in the way of these statements fulfilling themselves in your life.

Some Pregnancy Affirmations

My body is beautiful and strong.
My baby is growing, beautiful and strong.
I am and will be a good parent to my child (children).
The Universe loves and supports me and my baby.
My baby and I are ready for the Divine Plan of our lives to unfold.

The baby is naturally developing and doing just what it should.
Pregnancy is natural, normal, healthy, safe and divine for me and my baby.

Some Birth Affirmations

My body knows how to give birth and I will let it.
Contractions help my baby to be born.
Strong contractions are good ones.
I am strong and I can let my contractions be strong.
I am calm and relaxed. My baby feels my calmness and shares it.
The baby and I are rested and ready for the work we will do.
With each contraction my cervix is dilating a little more.
My contractions are massaging the baby and hugging it.
The baby is descending naturally. The baby's head fits perfectly in my pelvis.
I am opening.
I accept the healthy pain of labor, if and when it is here.
I feel the love of those who are helping me.
I send love to my baby and call him or her to my arms.

Some Postpartum Affirmations

My body is beautiful and strong.
My body knows how to make milk and nurse my baby and I will let it.
I am adjusting to life with my new baby.
I share in the strength and wisdom of all mothers.

The following suggestions for ways of working with affirmations come from Informed Birth and Parenting instructor Peg Merrill:

Probably the simplest and most effective way to work with affirmations is to write each one ten or twenty times on a sheet of paper, leaving a space in the right-hand margin of the page for the "emotional response." As the affirmation is written on the left side of the page, jot down whatever thoughts, considerations, beliefs, fears, or emotions come to your mind. Keep repeating the affirmation and notice how the responses on the right side change.

Here are some other suggestions of hers for working with affirmations:

1. Work with one or more every day. The best times are just before sleeping, before starting the day, or when you are feeling troubled.

2. Write each affirmation ten or twenty times with a response column. Writing is an extremely powerful technique of auto-suggestion.

3. Put specific names and situations into the affirmation. Include your name in the affirmation. Say and write each affirmation in the first, second, and third person — I (*Your Name*) love myself; You, (*Name*), love yourself; (*Name*) now loves herself.

4. Play with the vocabulary in the affirmation — make it personal and meaningful to yourself. Be specific about your desired result.

5. Record your affirmations on cassette tapes and play them back when you can. A good time is while driving or when going to bed. If you fall asleep it will still work!

6. Try looking into the mirror and saying the affirmations to yourself out loud. Keep saying them until you are able to see yourself with a relaxed, happy expression. Keep saying them until you eliminate all facial tension and grimaces.

7. Sit across from a partner, each of you in a straight chair, with your hands on your thighs and knees barely touching. Say the affirmation to your partner until you are comfortable doing it. Your partner can observe your body language carefully; if you squirm, fidget, or are unclear, you do not pass. He or she should not allow you to go on until you say it very clearly without contrary body reactions and upsets. Then your partner says them back to you, using the second person and your name. This continues until you can receive them without embarrassment. This is harder than it sounds!

8. Don't give up! If you ever get to a point where you begin to feel upset, shaky or afraid about something negative you discover, don't panic. Keep on writing the applicable affirmation over and over until your mind takes on the new thought. As it does, the negativity will fall away and you will feel lighter and better. Remember, it is just as easy to think positively as negatively. In fact it is easier. Negative thinking actually takes more effort.

9. Don't be afraid to experiment. Affirmations can be useful in all areas of your life—for problems at work, problems with health, personal growth, any problems at all.

Pregnancy is a time of heightened relationship. Values and beliefs get called into question as everything must make room for this new being. We hope that your relationships with your family and your inner self will deepen during this time. Growth is not always easy or painless, but it is fulfilling.

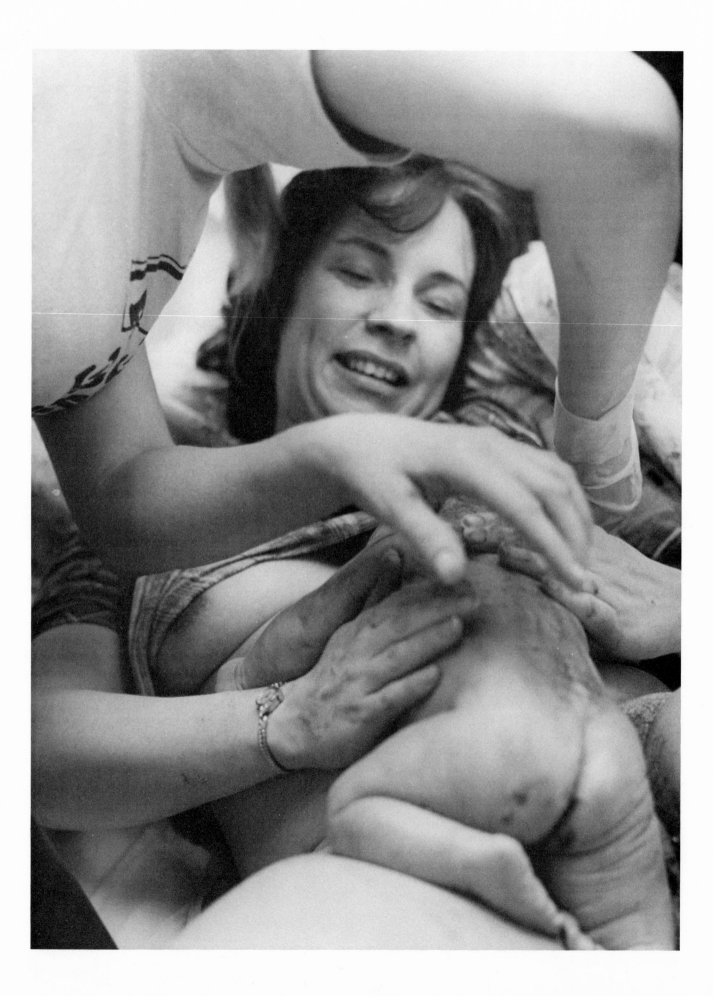

8
Looking Toward Giving Birth

While no one can really provide an adequate picture of labor and delivery for someone who has never given birth, you can do many things to increase your knowledge, relaxation, confidence, openness, and joy during labor and delivery.

The single most important key to a positive experience is relaxation. If it were possible to hold our arm muscles tense for eleven hours, we would be in great pain from lactic acid buildup. The uterine muscles wisely have the sense to contract and release in an effective and rhythmic pattern. But tension in our minds and lower bellies or shoulders during labor can actually cause a great deal of unnecessary suffering and slow down the course of labor.

We need to become confident that our body, just as it has known how to grow a baby, knows how to give birth. "As we trust the flowers to open, so can we trust birth" is the message on a beautiful poster of opening peonies by midwife/photographer Harriette Hartigan. Dr. Michel Odent speaks of the importance of the environment in encouraging women to get into their "instinctual selves." When a woman is relaxed and uninterrupted by bright lights, changing staff, and frequent pelvic exams, it is easier for her body to maintain the optimal levels of oxytocin and pain-relieving endorphins that lead to an unmedicated and satisfying delivery.

A woman who has given birth tends to have more confidence and security than a first-time mother. She has been through it all once before, knows what it felt like and knows that she can do it. But she can't really know what *this* labor and delivery will be like. This is partly because every labor is different, but also because giving birth is of a different order of magnitude from ordinary experiences. It's hard for one state of consciousness to remember another; it is only possible to remember *that it occurred* or to have tastes of it (flashbacks). A woman having her fifth baby was surprised by the intensity and said while in labor, "Now I remember what it felt like." It must also be added that the body produces its own endorphins during labor, chemicals that decrease pain and the memory of it and euphorically alter the woman's state of consciousness.

Fear is a natural part of contemplating giving birth, because birth is so momentous and has the element of the unknown about it. There is a normal element of fear a person feels before the wedding (the jitters) or before surgery. You'd be abnormal if you didn't feel afraid, or at least have moments of apprehension and doubt about going through labor and delivery. But fear can be reduced to a manageable level by clearing the past, acquiring knowledge and confidence about your ability to give birth and handle the intensity of contractions, and creating a supportive situation in which to birth.

Becoming Informed
Self-Education

Educating oneself about pregnancy, childbirth and parenting is an effective way to dispel fears and uncertainties, as well as supplying information to help make important decisions. Experience *is* the best teacher—it is a mistake to rely too much on books and the advice of others. However, having a sound basis of facts can help one to make wiser decisions.

Not knowing *how* your body gives birth leads to fear of the process, which causes tension. Tension, or tightening of the muscles, causes pain, which reinforces the fear and creates more tension until your body and psyche are exhausted. Your heart and uterine muscles, by contrast, work rhythmically through contraction and release and can easily work for many hours without tiring. The uterus knows its work, and if you can relax and let that happen, without tightening stomach or shoulders or the circular muscles that hold the uterus closed, labor will

progress with the minimum amount of effort and pain.

Knowledge can also help you to retain your decision-making ability in the face of minor complications. Like a road map, an understanding of the signs of early and advanced labor can help you know where you are when you reach them.

Educational sources include friends and family, classes, books, and experience. One must temper personal advice of family and friends with the knowledge that it is based on what happened to one other individual and thus may not relate exactly to your own particular and unique situation. Advice may, however, inspire you to seek more information or make a decision.

Special Delivery was written to provide parents with information about pregnancy, normal labor and delivery, and complications, so they would be able to maintain responsibility and make informed decisions. It takes the viewpoint that parents want this level of understanding and responsibility and are able to understand what is happening to their bodies and their baby. Because pregnancy and birth are described in detail in *Special Delivery,* we will not deal with them here. (Other helpful books can be found listed in the Appendix of this work.)

Most communities offer classes related to pregnancy, birth and parenting. Often doctors and midwives have practical classes available for their pregnant clients. But see that their classes are oriented toward choices, not just a description of their own particular practice. The local American Red Cross chapter may offer parenting classes. Another source of classes may be the local women's center and/or alternative educational institutions. La Leche League offers classes and information concerning breast-feeding and LLL volunteers are often good sources of information about the community birthing scene as well. Where classes on alternatives are not available, you can use the Informed Homebirth Tape Series of twelve lessons by Rahima Baldwin, or you can train to become a childbirth educator and start teaching.[1] There are many groups that offer teacher training, some of which are listed in the Appendix under "Resource Addresses."

The experience of being at a birth may be difficult to obtain before you have your child. Reading, seeing movies and slides, hearing other people's stories about pregnancy, birth and parenting can provide vicarious experience. You can imagine that the same circumstances are happening to you, and then experience your feelings, thoughts, and impulses to action, but they obviously aren't the real thing.

Support Groups

Support groups are essential for most people. They can be as informal as friends, or as structured as specialized groups that meet for specific support purposes. In this time of mobility, the need for specific support groups has increased.

Support groups offer a chance to learn how others deal with a situation similar to yours, to share emotional support, and to realize that others have survived what you are going through. The groups often offer specific educational information, as well as referrals.

When a situation is really overwhelming or too painful, please get in touch with a mental health care provider. He or she can offer a fresh perspective as well as useful techniques to deal with the difficulties.

Some Possible Sources of Support

women's consciousness raising groups	friends/family
parenting groups	childbirth educators
mothers' groups	church groups
childbirth classmates	midwives/doctors
C/sec (dealing with cesarean birth)	prenatal exercise classmates
La Leche League (for breastfeeding)	mental health center
Parents Anonymous (child abuse)	March of Dimes (birth defects)
Cesarean Prevention Movement (on vaginal birth after cesarean)	Mothers of Twins
	Parents Without Partners
	Hospice (for grieving families)

Childbirth Preparation Classes—Going Beyond Technique

Childbirth preparation classes are an excellent opportunity for you and your partner to focus together on the pregnancy and birth. This is their primary value for second- or third-time parents, who may have the knowledge of what will happen but lack the time and intimacy to focus on this particular pregnancy the way they need to. For first-time parents, classes are invaluable for the information, visual aids and interactive support they provide.

Most people have heard of Lamaze classes and many have heard of the Bradley Method. These are very valuable, but so are classes by instructors who take a more eclectic approach and don't teach any one method. Such instructors usually receive training through organizations such as the International Childbirth Educational Association (ICEA) or Informed Birth and Parenting (IH/IBP). There is no need to feel insecure if you don't learn a method with someone's name attached to it because methods are not the essential ingredient for giving birth with consciousness and joy. Tools for relaxation, communication and comfort are included in all good classes. They should help you to gain confidence in your own inner strength and ability to give birth, rather than teach methods that are to be followed by rote.

When investigating childbirth preparation classes, ask if techniques include a set breathing pattern and encourage you to get away from sensation, or if they encourage you to relax and breathe through the sensations. Ask what books are used or recommended. Ask to what extent cesarean prevention is discussed. Ask if there is any discussion of psychological aspects. Ask if the instructor works for a doctor or hospital or if she works privately, in which case classes are more likely to be choice-oriented. Ask about the instructor's own births and professional training.

Informed Homebirth/Informed Birth and Parenting instructors have been trained in a program developed by Rahima which uses both *Special Delivery* and this book for class reading, with an emphasis on class discussion and interaction that cannot be gained from books. For referral to instructors near you, write IH/IBP, Box 3675, Ann Arbor, MI 48106. Many other national organizations and private instructors also offer consumer oriented childbirth classes. See the Appendix for their addresses.

Childbirth preparation classes are invaluable for men, who are often excited about the possibility of seeing their baby born, but tend to know even less about birth than their wives. They can be apprehensive about the responsibility, or about what their role should be. If your husband is going to help you to be as comfortable as possible during labor and to stay centered during contractions, he needs to know what will be happening and what he can best do to help. He also needs to understand complications, various options, the side effects of anesthesia, and so on, since he will be involved in decision-making in the event of complications and may be called upon to act as your advocate.

If your husband is reluctant to become involved in the birth, childbirth preparation classes will often change his mind. Many times the husband who sits by the door, there only to fulfill his responsibility, turns out to be the most excited by the end of the series, when he has seen other men in that context and understands what his role can be. If your husband is adamant about not wanting to be at the birth, you can either resent or accept him for being who he is. But in either case you need to be active in finding someone else (friend, mother, sister) to be your labor assistant. Have this person attend classes with you and prepare together so she knows what is important to you during the birth.

Breathing and Relaxation

Relaxation is the key to labor, and ways of achieving that state have been discussed in the preceding chapter and in *Special Delivery*. Focused breathing encourages relaxation and keeps your attention on something besides your uterus. Elizabeth Noble in *Childbirth with Insight*[2] reminds us that "normal" breathing can vary from 5 to 20 breaths/minute according to the woman; conforming to a fixed pattern is not only unphysiological, but can lead to hyperventilation in the woman or hypoxia in the baby. Relaxing, consciously breathing with each contraction, and opening are conscious choices that can be made with each contraction. We recommend deep abdominal breathing because it is the normal breathing of relaxation (watch your partner's or child's breathing as he falls asleep). It is a tremendous experience to be filled with the power of creation; opening to it, breathing through it, and remaining in contact with your own strength and the support of your partner or assistant can turn birth from something painful and scary to an exhilarating and powerful event that transforms all who are present.

Dreams and Realities:
The Ideal and the Real

Put yourself in a relaxed state and visualize an ideally supportive birth situation. Let the environment be just right and imagine those people present who would be most supportive to you. Imagine the experience of labor and birth and holding your new baby. Then write down your ideal birth experience as you just visualized it—what happened, who was there, where it occurred, what you gained from it. Be sure to date it, and compare it with similar visualizations at various times in your pregnancy.

We all share such dreams and longings. Making them conscious can be helpful. You may want to share your vision with your partner and compare it with his expectations. Follow up on your ideal birth image by imagining yourself as an ideal parent— your philosophy of childcare, your routine, special little things that you will do for your child, how your life will change as the child grows.

The word *ideal* means "1. Conforming to an ultimate form of perfection or excellence. 2. Considered the best of its kind. 3. Completely or highly satisfactory. 4. Existing only in the mind; visionary; imaginary. 5. Of, pertaining to, or consisting of ideas or mental images."[3] The ideal is a model for our minds to work with and work towards. Few things, if any, in this material world are totally perfect. Yet everything has its own perfection, as an individual or experience that can never be exactly duplicated and as the lesson we need to confront at that moment of time. Each situation also provides the opportunity to fulfill a higher ideal—to positively make the best of everything one encounters in life.

Ideals can lead to disappointment when we do not remember that they are not fixed entities, and that they are seldom totally realized. You may have discovered this in your relationship with your partner. Your original ideal of a relationship might not be fulfilled. However, you have seen the real advantages and good points of what you have, and learned to cope with those things that are not ideal. Perhaps you have even altered your ideal partner-image after being with your real partner. A similar process may occur with your pregnancy, birth, and childcare experience. And if your baby doesn't look or act like your ideal baby, it may take you a while to get used to that and to know and love your child as a real individual.

Active Visualization of Normal Labor and Delivery

If it is impossible to practice giving birth, it *is* possible to educate more than your mind about the process. For example, listening to a tape recording of a birth can engage your emotions and the body reactions such emotions evoke. This kind of learning works into your body and your unconscious mind in a way the written word cannot touch.

Visualizations can work similarly by bypassing our rational minds, which are ready to understand and categorize birth, but which are inadequate to the task of birthing when it occurs. When visualizations are led by another person who is skilled in voice modulations, they can evoke reactions similar to those caused by real contractions. Thus the body can begin to experience its automatic tensing reaction followed by your conscious relaxation during a contraction and the great release when a contraction is over, even though you may never have experienced real contractions.

To do this active visualization of a normal labor and delivery, you can either have someone read it aloud or pre-record it on a tape for playback while you are in a state of deep relaxation. Alter particular facts to fit your birthing situation—birth place, plan, attendants. The reader should go slowly when talking about relaxation, increasing in tempo and intensity as the contractions build. Emphasize words that say what you are wanting, such as *release, down,* and *open.*

Let yourself completely relax by deepening your breathing. Feel as if your whole body is heavy, sinking down into thick, luxurious carpeting or sand at the beach. Let any thoughts or concerns of the day leave you on your breath. Now feel any tension you might have in your shoulders and let it go down and out your arms, so they lie relaxed and loose. Let your stomach be released, rising and falling as you breathe, and imagine any tension there going out with your breath. Let any tension from your buttocks and thighs flow down and out your legs. You don't need that tension, and your legs don't need to support you now.

With your mind's eye, travel to the back of your neck and around your eyes, letting any tension fall away on the lines of your hair. Just let it fall completely away. Feel your throat loose and relaxed,

and imagine the air coming in your throat and going all the way down to your vagina, gently surrounding and cradling your baby.

Now let yourself imagine what your baby might look like on the inside, floating in the waters, gently rocked by your breathing and soothed by the beating of your heart.

Men, imagine a window through which you can see your baby, healthy and growing inside your partner. Let yourself imagine the red walls of the uterus, firmly supporting your baby, and the placenta, so dark and healthy with its two arteries and vein in the cord.

Just as your body knows how to nourish and support your baby through the placenta, it also knows how to give birth. And just as your inner organs have changed to make room for the growing baby, so an inner growth or learning that needs to take place will do so naturally, without any effort on your part.

Now imagine a day in the future when it will be the perfect time for your labor to begin. You have been feeling an intermittent tightening in your lower belly, not unlike the contractions you have often felt during the last few weeks of your pregnancy. But as the contractions become more regular and more intense, you realize you are in early labor. Your body and baby have begun the process of birth, just as nature intended.

You talk to your baby, telling it how happy you are that you will soon see each other and touch skin-to-skin. You have told your partner and birth attendant, and now you decide to go for a walk or continue your normal activities, breathing through the contractions as necessary. If it is night, you go back to sleep until contractions wake you with their growing strength. (Pause)

Now you feel a contraction growing and building, like the sound of a train approaching from far away, getting stronger and more intense, building until it is right upon you. Then it slowly fades as it goes off into the distance. And you rest between contractions as the natural process of labor continues, perfected through countless generations of women. (Pause)

As you feel the next contraction starting to build, you open to what your body genetically and instinctively knows, letting it build and build, feeling it become harder and stronger as you welcome its increasing intensity. You hear your deep and steady breathing as the contraction builds toward the peak . . . and then gradually eases off and fades away. And you rest, calling on the vast source of inner strength that is available to you. (Pause)

Now you feel another contraction starting to build, like a wave that builds and builds and finally peaks before sliding in to shore. And you feel a gush as your own waters break and flow out, warm between your legs. And you rest, and your baby rests, being massaged and prepared for birth by your strong and effective contractions. (Pause)

And now, as you feel an intense contraction that nearly takes your breath away, you surrender to its power and imagine it opening your cervix right over your baby's head. You allow this energy of birth to flow through you, like water through a channel, a clear, open channel for the birth of your baby. And then you rest, gathering your strength for the next contraction. (Pause)

The sensation builds rapidly again, and you open, visualizing your baby's head sliding right down through the circle of your open cervix. You are one with your contractions, their rhythm is yours, and you dance with them. You release everything to the power of these contractions, which now seem back-to-back. You feel the love and support of your partner and attendants and you feel your connection with all women as you open to the energy of birth. And then the contraction fades away, and you rest, and your baby rests, preparing for the journey of birth. (Pause)

As the next contraction starts to build, you call on your inner strength and courage. You remember your baby who is working to find the perfect pathway through your birth canal, into your loving arms. As the contraction builds, you feel as if you need to have a bowel movement. But it is the baby you feel, soon to come out. You breathe through this new sensation and feel excitement and new energy filling you as you realize your baby is starting to descend. (Pause.)

Now you are completely open as the next contraction builds and builds, surging through you. You help the natural pushing of your uterus by your own efforts. You take several deep breaths, almost as though you are in the excitement of making love. Then you direct your energy downward and outward, opening like a rose, relaxing your vagina and perineum to let the fruit of your love flow out. Your throat and face are relaxed, your chin down on your chest, your legs open and floppy. As the contraction subsides, you breathe deeply

and relax totally, giving yourself and the baby plenty of oxygen. (Pause)

You tell the baby how much you want to see her or him and that it won't be long now. The next contraction swells and builds with that catch in your throat, and you feel the baby come down as you completely open down below. You surrender to the intensity and let it happen. You let your strong uterus push your baby out. Your face and throat, like your pelvic floor and perineum, are loose and relaxed. Your muscles stretch naturally over your baby's head. (Pause)

You completely relax between contractions, and your birth attendant begins to massage your supple perineum, helping it to stretch easily. And now as the contraction builds, more of your baby's head is visible as it plunges down and stretches the opening of your vagina. And you let it happen, opening completely. And the contraction fades, and you rest. (Pause)

The contraction builds again and you feel a stinging sensation as your healthy skin stretches to let your baby out. You know that the baby is close to crowning. You breathe through the contraction and touch your baby's head as your birth attendant supports your perineum. You open with the contraction and then relax totally as it subsides. (Pause)

As the next contraction builds, you breathe through it while your birth attendant gently guides your baby's head out without tearing. The sensation is intense, and so is the release once the head is born. Feeling excited, you wait for the next contraction while your baby is suspended between two worlds, not yet born and yet no longer fetus.

After two or three timeless minutes another strong contraction comes and births your baby completely. You reach down and touch the baby as it is brought up onto your chest. Your baby breathes and pinks up immediately, having been massaged and prepared for birth by the strong contractions of your uterus. As you gaze into the eyes of your newborn for the first time, you are lost for a moment in their depths. Allow yourself to imagine what it will be like for the two of you, holding your new baby for the first time. (Long pause)

You put your baby to your breast and, after a few preliminary licks and tastes, he or she latches on and begins to suck. You feel a contraction again and hand your husband the baby, whose cord has been cut after it stopped pulsing. Your placenta comes completely loose from your uterus and is *pushed out naturally. Your uterus continues to contract firmly with minimal loss of blood. You give thanks for the miracle of birth, and take this time to share together as a new family.* (Pause)

And now let this vision fade into the future, to the time your body knows is right for your baby to be born. And turn your attention now to your baby in your current state of pregnancy, floating in the waters, protected, healthy, growing. Feel your body, which knows how to grow this baby, and feel that any changes or learning that need to take place will do so naturally without your having to worry about it, for your body knows how to give birth.

Now feel your arms and legs, moving your feet and hands as you become aware of the room in which you are lying and slowly open your eyes, feeling relaxed and refreshed.

What was your experience of the above visualization? Lead your partner through it too, having him imagine a window into your uterus. Change the visualization to make it smoother for you. Did you feel that your body was adapting and learning without your conscious effort? For further work with visualizations for special situations or fears, see *Birthing Normally* by Gayle Peterson.[4]

Dealing with Fear and Pain

Pain

Pain has not been a popular word among childbirth educators. It is unfashionable to have pains during childbirth. Instead, we have "intense sensations," or "rushes," or the emotionlessly named "contractions." These at least give us more freedom of interpretation than having "pains," but what if it hurts? Certainly, some women may not experience their labor as painful, but others do. As one friend told us, following a beautiful, natural delivery in a birthing center, "No one can tell me those weren't pains!" Neither feeling nor not feeling pain during labor is "right" or more natural. Each is a unique experience of the birthing process. Each woman's body, pain threshold, expectations, size and position of the baby, preparation for the birth, and many other factors enter into those experiences and how they are interpreted.

By denying the possibility of some pain in labor we may be forced either to deny our own sensations or to believe that there is something wrong with us or what we are doing. Such a situation may also lead a woman to hold back her contractions because she's not sure that she can stand them getting stronger without admitting that it hurts, resulting in a longer and possibly ineffective labor.

There may be times in labor when it seems impossible to be comfortable. Being able to experience this, and then keep on with whatever needs to be done, can greatly smooth the way of the birth.

We believe that all of the playing down of the possibility of pain in labor is a reaction to the stories of fearful, screaming women agonizing in labor, and to the biblical reference that all women must experience pain during childbirth. It is done in an attempt to calm the fears of women that the pain will be too much to bear, especially if they are hoping for a natural birth without any "painkillers."

We feel it is more helpful to foster an attitude of self-confidence and strength to withstand any necessary pain, while releasing tension to prevent any unnecessary pain. This takes conscious effort on the part of women who have grown up in a society where females are labeled weak and helpless, and where we are encouraged to rid ourselves of every little ache and pain with some type of drug rather than by self-sufficient means.

Some Self-Evaluation Concerning Pain

Do you consider yourself to be chicken, macho, or normal when it comes to withstanding physical pain?

_____

_____

_____

On what do you base this self-image?

_____

_____

_____

_____

What is the most physically painful memory that you have?

_____

_____

_____

What did you do with the pain?

_____

_____

_____

Have you ever healed yourself of a pain naturally?

_____

_____

_____

When you were a child, how did your parents react when you hurt yourself?

_____

_____

_____

Do you now react the same way or differently?

_____

_____

_____

Most of us deal with pain and discomfort in our birthings according to our approach to life. The passive approach is to "take something for it." The active approach is to use relaxation, visualization, affirmation, and preventive measures to take care of as much of the pain as possible. Since no medication has been proven totally safe for the baby before or during labor, the active approach seems

better for the little one. It also allows more active participation by the mother in the labor and the birth, leading to more effective work, more personal satisfaction, and fewer interventions to compensate for a numb or half-conscious mother.

Active Pain Relief Techniques for Labor

1. *Relaxation.* Practice can help make relaxation a reflex (see Touch Relaxation, Chapter 7).
2. *Visualization.* Try seeing and feeling the painful area opening, relaxing, getting warmer and more fluid, filling with light.
3. *Remember the baby.* Say "I love you, baby" and tell him or her that soon you will see each other.
4. *Affirmation.* "I let go of this sensation that has taught me to relax even more." "I am stronger than this sensation and can let it be, without fighting it." "I release this pain to Mother Earth (or to the Infinite One, to God)."
5. *Massage.* You can massage yourself or ask your partner or other attendant to assist you.
6. *Preventive techniques.* Rest toward the end of your pregnancy to prevent over-fatigue during labor; eat easily digestible foods in early labor and drink energy-giving liquids throughout labor; verbalize worries so they can be dealt with and do not aggravate sensations; be self-confident and knowledgeable about the process of birth; try changing your position during labor to find what is comfortable; have positive, loving people around you.

Fear

We have discussed that a general fear of the unknown is normal and even healthy. Most fear is oriented toward the future, influenced by past experiences of pain or loss that you are afraid will occur again. Fear in the present moment occurs when the body alerts us or we otherwise realize that there is danger. Then the fight or flight mechanism is activated to get us out of that situation.

During childbirth, however, we must consciously *override* any bodily fear reactions. It isn't effective to deny them, and it's probably impossible to completely eliminate them. The body experiences pain and tenses up, getting ready to get you out of there. You need to tell the body, "Thank you very much. I got the message. But we're going to stay right here. This sensation is all right." This is a time when the body's reaction is counterproductive. Fear removed from any present-time danger can be seen as a discordant expression of safety energy. Therefore, it is appropriate to use it as a guide to those areas where you have a wish or need for safety. The following steps, based on work by Juana Bordas, MSW, Director of MiCasa Resource Center for Women in Denver, will help you to do just that:

1. Name your fears about pregnancy, childbirth and parenting here. Besides writing them down, talk with someone about them, to get them out in the open. Look at your dreams, too.

Some common fears include: death of self or baby; pain; deformity; loss of self-identity in the mothering role; inability to be a good parent; inability to provide financially for one's child(ren); the possibility of episiotomy, drugs, forceps, or cesarean during the birth.

2. Find out the facts concerning the likelihood and circumstances that would lead to each fear being realized.

3. Name possible and probable results if that fear were realized.

4. Name and take steps to avoid the fear being realized, based on the information you learned in step two. Decide the steps you would take, if the fear were realized, to make the best of the situation.

5. Affirm your work on the fear. If it continues to plague you emotionally after you have taken the suggested steps, then begin consciously to drain the fear of its energy. Since you have already acted on the fear in a positive way, this is different from repression. Here are some methods to help defuse a fear you have already evaluated and worked on:

● **When the fear arises, tell it, "I no longer need to hear you. I have already done all I can to prevent your realization and have accepted you as a possibility that I can face, if realized."**
● **Tell the fear, "I have done my part to be safe and I now have faith in nature (or God) that all will work out for my eventual betterment."**
● **Do relaxation exercises while doing an affirmation such as the preceding two.**
● **Do progressive desensitization, which follows.**

Progressive Desensitization

Progressive desensitization is a technique for getting rid of excess emotion connected to a given situation. It is useful for when you have recognized the emotion and its reason for existence and then done everything possible to alleviate the need for that emotion.

Take for example, the fear of having a deformed baby. Nightmares or a magazine article may bring this fear to awareness. It can then be used as motivation to do everything you can to have a healthy baby by learning what can prevent deformity. After learning and doing everything possible to prevent the realization of this fear, some fear may still remain. Since that fear is no longer useful, try progressive desensitization.

1. Sit down and objectively list different situations or things that elicit the emotion you are working on ranging from the least intense for you to handle, to the most intense (e.g. birthmark, missing toes, cleft lip, heart murmur . . .).

2. Get into a state of deep relaxation.

3. Start with the least difficult item on your list. Imagine it, while staying totally relaxed, without putting any emotion into it. Say an appropriate affirmation. See the situation now at its best. Go on to the next level of intensity, and continue *only* as long as you can remain totally relaxed. What you are doing is relearning a response to a situation. (For example, imagine the baby has a birthmark. Stay totally relaxed, seeing the baby with love. Repeat, "I am doing my best to help my baby form whole and healthy." Now, see the baby totally normal. Go on to the next level.)

Various Women's Dialogues with Birthing Energy (B.E.)

> *Me:* *I'm afraid. I don't think that I'll be able to relax.*
> *B.E.:* *Don't worry. I'll help you. I'll give you the strength. I'll give you courage. Hold on, you'll be OK.*
> *Me:* *No. I'm afraid to let go. I'm afraid that I'll go to pieces. Will I be able to take it?*

B.E.: Of course you'll be able to take it. Just relax and let yourself go. Now take some nice deep breaths and relax your body completely. Relax yourself completely. When you feel your uterus tightening up, let go completely.

Me: Who are you?

B.E.: I am the energy of your birth.

Me: Well, you hurt.

B.E.: Yes, but you will be able to handle it.

Me: How will you feel?

B.E.: I will feel different at different times.

Me: How can I work with you?

B.E.: You should not tense up—just move with me. Be flexible. Don't have a set part. Just read me as I happen.

Me: (not pregnant): I am afraid you will be more than I can handle.

B.E.: You are afraid of being afraid.

Me: That's true. But I know you are so powerful!

B.E.: I am powerful—and you can be a channel.

Me: That makes me feel better. I am part of me wanting to experience you again but feel that this is not the right time.

B.E.: That's all right, you can use me when it is time.

Me: In the meantime, I want to keep an awareness of you and how to flow with you so that I can help other women in their births.

B.E.: I am not to be feared. I am very strong. I am the power that transforms.

Me: Many of us fear that change. Anticipating changing your life is scary.

B.E.: But when you relax and let yourself go, you allow yourself to change, to grow, to go on to the next place.

Me: Dear Birthing Energy, I fear you are stronger. Will I handle myself in the correct manner?

B.E.: Dear Me, you are strong by right, and we are one. You are part of all that is. Do not fear. Even the tiger has no room to insert its fierce claws. You are protected!

Me: But how will/can I find this protection? Where?

B.E.: You have only to experience your inner self.

B.E.: Well, Joan, I think we're going to be working together soon and I think it's going to be a good learning experience for both of us.

Me: Yeah, I think I know you a bit more than last time. I think I trust myself more this time, so I'll be able to trust you. And I'm expecting to learn a lot more about you next time around. I almost feel that you are a part of me right now. Not just something separate, an idea, philosophy . . .

B.E.: Yeah, I think I'm gonna surprise you.

Me: I'm sure you will!

Fear of Dying

It is ironic that the process of birthing a new life puts us closely in touch with death—yet both are transitions into and out of this earthly life. The possibility of our death is always with us. Now is an opportunity to acknowledge death as a contributor to our lives. It can keep us honest and in the moment.

This exercise may bring up a lot of emotions. Please do not avoid them—deal with them. After finishing, or after any question you find particularly distressing, relax and visualize you and your family together, healthy, and happy.

● **What do I believe happens to a person after death?**

_____

_____

_____

_____

● **What does my partner believe?**

_____

_____

_____

● If I die, what details will my partner need to deal with? What can I do now to help make it easier (e.g. a will, a last letter, a discussion about what kind of burial and funeral you prefer.)?

_____

_____

_____

_____

_____

● What if the baby dies? What details would we need to deal with (e.g. bonding, naming, autopsy, funeral, burial.)?

_____

_____

_____

_____

_____

There may be a local hospice organization with support groups for those who are grieving for a baby or other family member who has died. They could also provide information concerning choices and procedures.

Once, After Reading About Buddha Sending His Student To Watch the Constant Burning of The Dead at the Funeral Pyres, as a Lesson in the Inevitability of Death . . .

*when the Teacher speaks of Death
I am so afraid that I eat 17 peanut butter cookies, fall down, shivering, and kiss the floor, and quickly write something down, hoping that I won't really disappear.*

Terra

Fear of Episiotomy or Tearing

With no intention of going from the sublime to the ridiculous, we want to follow fear of dying by discussing fear of tearing or having an episiotomy (a cut made in the area between the vagina and the anus to increase the size of the vaginal opening). We have found that more women fear tearing or being cut than are afraid of dying in childbirth. While few women die in childbirth in this country, 95 percent of all birthing women have an episiotomy, and a sizeable percentage of those birthing with perineal support do in fact tear. These facts, combined with our inability to imagine how a head so big can come out of a hole so small, make this a topic worth addressing. No woman wants her genitals cut or wants the discomfort of stitches postpartum if they can be avoided.

Abundant studies show that routine episiotomy has no beneficial effects on the pelvic floor.[5] Show them to your doctor, but unless he has worked with midwives, he probably doesn't know how to deliver with perineal support (it's not taught in medical school). Also, perineal support involves the potential for "success or failure" in a way which an episiotomy doesn't, so it's more of a threat to him.

An episiotomy is only necessary on the rare occasions when a distressed infant needs to be gotten out quickly. Otherwise you are better off delivering the head gradually while allowing your tissues to stretch. You may deliver without any tearing, and pelvic-floor exercises will return tone to your muscles. Even if you do tear, you will have torn at the weakest point in your tissues rather than having an episiotomy scar as well as the weakest point in future deliveries. Although scar tissue is stronger, the tissue next to it is more likely to tear. See *Special Delivery* for techniques of perineal support.

Some factors related to tearing or not tearing:

1. The condition of your tissues (good nutrition, including extra vitamins C and E, perineal massage, and pelvic floor exercises definitely help).
2. Your position during the late second stage (letting your legs flop apart, rather than imitating the stirrups position, aids in the relaxation of the pelvic floor; a straight squat is supposed to equalize pressure all around; the side position

lessens pressure on the perineum; hands-and-knees does too, but can result in more tears to the front).

3. How well you are able to stop pushing when the baby's head crowns.
4. The size and presentation of your baby's head.
5. The extent to which your birth attendants are able to help you with a gentle delivery of the head.

The positive approach to prevention:

1. Excellent nutrition.
2. Practice with second stage pushing and not-pushing. You might find out what different techniques are available by attending childbirth classes and/or reading books on the various methods. Pushing is really an involuntary reflex, like orgasm; avoid holding your breath and assuming positions that are unphysiological. Listen to your body!
3. Be sure your birth attendant knows how to do perineal massage, support and other techniques for gentle delivery of the head.
4. Be sure to do perineal massage on yourself or with your partner the last six weeks of your pregnancy.
5. Do at least 100 pelvic floor exercises per day.
6. Practice relaxing your pelvic floor at will.

Some Exercises for the Pelvic Floor Muscles:

These exercises are designed to help you distinguish and strengthen the pelvic floor muscles (refer also to *Special Delivery* for detailed drawings and explanations).

1. Pull in all the muscles between your legs without tensing your thighs or buttocks. Hold the muscles in for a count of five. Release and relax.

2. Draw in and tighten your anal sphincter without tensing the muscles around your vagina. Hold the muscles for a count of five. Now release and relax.

3. Tighten your vaginal muscles to a count of three as you inhale. Now exhale and relax the entire pelvic floor as you count to four. This has also been called the Kegel exercise, and should be done faithfully many times each day.

Prenatal Perineal Massage

Massaging the tissue of your perineum between the vagina and the anus during the last six weeks of pregnancy can help prevent tearing during the birth. Massaging oil into the tissue and stretching it can help create less resistance to the birth of the head, and also help you learn to relax the pelvic floor muscles.

1. You can do the massage yourself, using your thumbs, but it is probably easier in the last six weeks of pregnancy for your husband or partner to do this with you. Make sure your bladder is empty and that you are propped up comfortably. When first starting, you might find that a warm bath softens your tissues. Use a mirror the first few times so you can become thoroughly familiar with the area.
2. Massage a natural oil (Vitamin E, wheat germ, cocoa butter, or whatever feels best) into the tissues of the perineum and lower vaginal wall. Pay special attention to any scar tissue from previous episiotomies.
3. Then your partner can put both index fingers about 3 inches into the vagina and press downward toward the rectum. While maintaining steady pressure, the fingers can be moved upward along the sides of the vagina in a rhythmic "sling" type of movement.
4. As you massage each night, your tissue will relax and stretch. Have your coach gently stretch the vaginal opening as wide as possible each time until you feel a tingling or burning sensation that says "far enough!" This will help you recognize the time to stop pushing so that the crowning head can slip out gently.
5. Hold this stretch, without hurting the mother, for a minute or two, then release. Massage with more oil, stretch again to the maximum, hold, and then release.
6. If you do this massage faithfully, your partner will be able to insert more fingers and perhaps his whole fist as you approach your due date and your perineum becomes more elastic. This assures that your tissues are supple and creates the confidence that a baby's head can surely fit through. It also reassures you that during the last month of pregnancy, the hormone *relaxin* is working in your body, helping your tissues and the ligaments of your pelvis to stretch and open naturally for labor and delivery.
7. Do a contraction of the vaginal muscle and feel where the PCG muscle lies and how strong it is. Feel how difficult stretching is when you are

tensing the muscles of the pelvic floor, and consciously release them as your coach does the stretching (hint: keep your mouth and throat really loose during the massage). By doing the pelvic-floor exercises after the birth, your muscles will regain their tone.

Women and midwives who make use of this stretching during the last month of pregnancy find it really helpful in preventing tearing. (For instructions on perineal massage and support during the delivery, see pages 65–66 in *Special Delivery*.)

Creating Your Own Birth Experience

Choices in Childbirth

Let us turn now from the inner feelings that you may have about birthing to the immediate environment in which you will give birth. Will you have your baby in the hospital or at home? Would you prefer a birth center? What does it offer that is unique? Will you birth with midwives, your doctor, or one of several doctors who might be on call? Will your husband be with you? What about your other children or a labor support person? What are your attendant's procedures and percentages regarding episiotomy, tearing or fetal monitoring? What kind of newborn exam is done? In the hospital, will you be able to have rooming-in? When will you go home? If birthing at home, what will your emergency back-up plan be?

Responsibility lies with you and your partner, as parents, to interview your doctor or midwife and know his or her procedures and limitations. It is impossible to compare births or to compare frameworks. The woman who says, "I hemorrhaged in the hospital. If I had been at home, I would have bled to death" is failing to realize that if she had been at home, she would have been quite a different person. Her nutrition during pregnancy might have been different, her attendants probably would have handled delivery of the placenta differently, she might not have bled at all, or it might have been handled by pitocin and/or transport to the hospital. Each birth is unique and can't be compared to any other.

The first step in creating what you want is knowing what you want, knowing what is important to you. Once you know, it may be easy to find the

attendants and setting that fit your needs. Or you may find you have to work very hard to create what you want. You may also find that your choices become more difficult if you are dealt physical factors such as a breech baby or bleeding during pregnancy. But making your own best choices at each step seems to be a real key to satisfaction with your birthing experience. To help in understanding what is important to you and your partner, try the following exercises.

What Do You Value?

Knowing what you value about pregnancy and birth can help you to act on the values and make them real, rather than unfulfilled wishes. On the following list underline the values you hold, rating the most important five, decreasing to one. Be sure to add any not listed.

Pregnancy Values

healthy mom	relaxation for mom
financial security	good prenatal care
relating to baby prenatally	childbirth classes
good sexual relationship with partner	healthy baby
	good nutrition
partner relates well to baby	prepare the layette
friends relate well to baby	regular exercise
your parents are happy	
other children relate well to baby	
Other ideas:	

Birthing Values

healthy baby	no tears or episiotomy
relaxed atmosphere	no IV or drugs
no medical problems	readily available emergency care
competent birth attendant	uninterrupted bonding
no psychological problems	control over environment
low financial cost	choosing labor and birth attendant
vaginal delivery	healthy mom
feeling no pain	familiar place
friends present	fast labor

partner present
siblings present
Other ideas:

father catches baby
latest medical equipment

Postpartum Values

baby with parents as
    much as possible
healthy mom
good nutrition
breastfeeding
stimulating environ-
    ment for baby
healthy dad
Other ideas:

sleep
financial security
healthy baby
stimulating environment
    for parents
safety
peace
support system

Issues of Pregnancy and Childbirth

There are many issues to consider and decisions to make concerning pregnancy and childbirth. This exercise will introduce some of them, so that you can see what you need to know more about, what you have already decided, and what you agree on with your partner. React to each with an agree (+), disagree (–), or undecided (?). Cover your reactions, ask your partner to do it, then compare.

Mother   Father

_____ _____ Prenatal care is important for a healthy mother and baby.

_____ _____ Hospitals are the best place to give birth.

_____ _____ Home birth can be safe with a skilled birth attendant.

_____ _____ The baby takes what it needs to grow from the mother.

_____ _____ There is no need to eat a special diet.

_____ _____ A woman's thoughts and feelings can affect her labor.

_____ _____ Sonograms are perfectly safe for pregnant mothers and their unborn babies.

Mother   Father

_____ _____ Alcohol, cigarette smoke, coffee, prescription and nonprescription drugs can all affect the unborn child.

_____ _____ Trained midwives are the best birth attendants for normal births.

_____ _____ Episiotomies are usually necessary.

_____ _____ Drugs given to the mother during labor adversely affect the baby.

_____ _____ Breathing and relaxation techniques are important to achieve an unmedicated birth

_____ _____ Cesarean sections can often be prevented by natural techniques.

_____ _____ Once a woman has had a cesarean she must always deliver her babies that way.

_____ _____ Eating and drinking during labor can cause problems.

_____ _____ Making sounds—even singing—during labor can help it progress.

_____ _____ Changing positions during labor is useful.

_____ _____ Walking during labor can be as helpful to its progress as using drugs like pitocin.

_____ _____ Babies need to be in an isolette right after they are born.

_____ _____ The placenta has to come out right away after the birth, even if the doctor must pull it out.

_____ _____ Fathers are not necessary at the birth.

_____ _____ Normal babies shouldn't be hung upside down and spanked right after they are born.

_____ _____ Babies should cry right after they are born.

_____ _____ Siblings should be allowed at the birth.

_____ _____ Pregnant women have the right to know the reason for, the effects of, and alternatives to any drugs or therapies offered to them.

The Place of Birth

Everyone puts the safety of mother and baby first in considering where they want to give birth. Some women feel safest in the hospital where the doctors' and nurses' experience and the presence of emergency equipment mean that no time need be lost in an emergency. Other women feel that the complications caused by a just-in-case philosophy and unnecessary equipment are a greater risk to their baby than the time spent in transport would be. They feel that their chances of having a normal birth are greater at home, and this outweighs the disadvantages of lack of equipment and the need to go to the hospital should major complications arise. Other women prefer a birth center, where they feel that doctors or midwives will treat them more as an individual while having emergency equipment immediately available.

The pros and cons of giving birth in a hospital, at home or in a birth center are numerous. Ultimately it must be the woman's and couple's decision. It is possible to have a safe and satisfying experience in any location. Understanding the procedures and limitations of your attendants and the location you choose can help you to make responsible decisions at each point along the way. Lack of communication is what leads to negative feelings and lawsuits. No one can guarantee the outcome of a birth. Saying "do it to me," whether to your obstetrician, midwife, or neighbor, invites disaster. Parents need to be involved in the decision-making process, because they need to live with the results for the rest of their lives.

Interviewing a Doctor

Many people are intimidated by interviewing a doctor. Doctors can seem so busy, and often annoyed, especially by someone who is "one of those consumer advocates." But there are an increasing number of doctors who will welcome your questions and approach, and if they don't take the time to find out what's important to you, your chances of getting it are not very great.

No one has unlimited resources, either financial or emotional, for interviewing doctors, but the investment is a vital one. You can make your task simpler by talking to other women (who share your values) about the experience they had with their doctor. One of the childbirth educators' most powerful tools is a file in which women write about their experience with their doctor. Then, without having to make politically touchy statements about any doctor, they can let the birthing women speak for themselves. Other childbirth educators will tell you straight out what your chances of having no anesthesia or a VBAC are with a certain doctor. La Leche League leaders also are great sources of information about who is really supporting women in birth in the community. Contacting your local chapter of the Cesarean Prevention Movement (or founding one) is also a sound bet. Or talk to women who have had a VBAC—a doctor who supports that is likely to be more supporting of women birthing with their own power.

When calling to make an appointment, ask for an interview. Trying to ask questions in a hospital gown while you're on the table puts you at an obvious disadvantage. Once you arrive and are introduced to one another, make a brief statement about your pregnancy and what is important to you in giving birth. Don't just hand him your 32 nonnegotiable demands to read! Lead from that into specific questions about his own attitudes and birthing practices. Ask specific questions that will give you interpretable answers, such as "What percentage of your women deliver without episiotomy?" rather than "When do you do an episiotomy?" ("Only when necessary," obviously; the fact that it's necessary 95 percent of the time escapes unnoticed.)

One primary concern should be whether this doctor will be at your delivery, or does he share a rotation with three or four associates? It's difficult to establish a relationship many times over, and doctors' views obviously differ, even within the same practice. If you will be seeing only one doctor, what happens if he is on vacation or not on call? How frequent is that, who covers for him, and do they respect his agreements or tend to follow differing views? Ask where he has hospital privileges, and whether the things you want would be possible there.

Doctors are at a disadvantage because most have had no training in communication or women's issues in medical school. Medical school, in fact, tends to be so gruelling that the only way they can survive a residency is to turn off their emotions and deny their own feelings. But you should at least feel comfortable with the man, as if you can talk and be heard. While it is fine to take your husband with you for these interviews, if you feel that you need a man present at every visit in order for the doctor to take your questions seriously, you may have the wrong doctor. The seeds of trust must be able to grow out of this first interview—not that you will trust him to "take care of everything," but that you can trust him to do what he says, to tell you what he wants to do, and to respect your participation in the decision-making process.

Don't forget that you are going into an agreement with a doctor to work *together*. A doctor can dismiss you from his care if he thinks you are lying to him or not following what he considers important health recommendations. And you can fire a doctor at any time, up to and including being in labor. As a health care consumer, you have the right to refuse treatment from anyone, even if you are in a hospital. Do your scouting as early in your pregnancy as possible, but if you find you have made the wrong decision, don't rule out other options, even late in your pregnancy.

Understanding the principles of informed consent can help you feel less at the mercy of the institution. The hospital requests that you sign a statement on admission giving blanket consent for all procedures. But you can amend this before signing it to read, "Providing each procedure is explained at the time and informed consent is given."

The American College of Obstetricians and Gynecologists has made a commendable effort to set forth clearly the patient's right of informed consent in the following excerpts from its *Standards of Obstetric-Gynecologic Services*.

It is important to note the distinction between consent and informed consent. Many physicians, because they do not realize there is a difference, believe they are free from liability if the patient consents to treatment. This is not true. The physician may still be liable if the patient's consent was not informed. In addition, the usual consent obtained by a hospital does not in any way release the physician from his legal duty of obtaining an informed consent from his patient.

Most courts consider that the patient is informed if the following information is given:

● *The processes contemplated by the physician as treatment, including whether the treatment is new or unusual.*
● *The risks and hazards of the treatment.*
● *The chances for recovery after treatment.*
● *The necessity of the treatment.*
● *The feasibility of alternative methods of treatment.*

One point on which courts do agree is that explanations must be given in such a way that the patient understands them. A physician cannot claim as a defense that he explained the procedure to the patient when he knew the patient did not understand. The physician has a duty to act with due care under the circumstances; this means he must be sure the patient understands what she is told.

It should be emphasized that the following reasons are not sufficient to justify failure to inform:

1. That the patient may prefer not to be told the unpleasant possibilities regarding the treatment.
2. That full disclosure might suggest infinite dangers to a patient with an active imagination, thereby causing her to refuse treatment.
3. That the patient, on learning the risks involved, might rationally decline treatment. The right to decline is the specific fundamental right protected by the informed consent doctrine.[6]

For more information, request "The Pregnant Patient's Bill of Rights and Responsibilities" available from the International Childbirth Education Association.[7]

Remember, too, that it is always possible to ask for a second opinion. Choose a doctor who is not in association with your physician. This will provide you with more data to use in making a decision. There are often several ways to treat something, so while one pediatrician may threaten child abuse charges if you don't put your baby in the hospital for treatment of jaundice, another may help you set up "bili lights" at home, and a third may prescribe another day of watching and waiting. You can dismiss one doctor and say you are going to use the services of another if need be.

Requests for Hospital Delivery

Before Rahima had her first child at home in 1973, she attended conventional Lamaze classes at a hospital and was as amazed to hear other people's birth plans as they were to hear hers. One woman said, "At my hospital, they keep the baby for twelve hours before letting you have it." Rahima expected the next sentence to be, "So we're changing hospitals.'' But that didn't happen. That's where their insurance put them, and that's just the way things were. Exercise your choice! You can change hospitals or doctors, or you can work to get what you want within the institution you have chosen! Your baby is only going to be born once. And *you* can't keep giving birth until you get it ''right.''

If you are going to give birth in the hospital, you need to know both your doctor's and the hospital's procedures. If you want something nonstandard, who has the higher authority, the doctor or the hospital? Each may say that the other won't allow it; in fact, the doctor can often get changes in standard procedure if they are requested in writing.

There are many things you can do during a hospital labor to keep from feeling weak or like a patient. Only sit in the wheelchair if you want to be waited on and get a free ride; beware of the danger of feeling sick and unable to do anything. Can you bypass such admission procedures as the shave and enema (this may have to be arranged in writing)? Can you pre-admit yourself so you and your husband won't need to be separated when you arrive at the hospital? Can you keep on your own clothing during labor? If you don't feel bold enough to wear a sexy negligee, even bringing a short smock with flowers on it would be an improvement over institutional taste in clothing! Donning the hospital gown makes you feel like a patient. No one needs to wear a gown in birth centers at hospitals, so what's the difference between your room and theirs?

To do your part in creating a birth experience with which you feel satisfied, make a list of requests for a hospital delivery. Even if you plan to have a home birth, make it clear in writing what you prefer if you do birth in the hospital. This will require that you first inform yourself about the options that are available. Arrange for a tour of the hospital. If no maternity open houses are scheduled, call the nurses on the night shift to see if you can come by sometime (the night shift tends to be younger, more liberal and less entrenched than those with seniority). Try to discuss all of your requests thoroughly with your doctor and/or birth attendants before birth time. Bring several copies of your requests with you if or when you go to the hospital so coach, nurses, and doctors will each have them handy for reference.

Here is a list of sample requests for hospital delivery that is used by teachers of Informed Birth and Parenting. It should be altered to suit your individual situation and preferences.

VAGINAL DELIVERY

1. Use of same room for labor and delivery.
2. Husband's and coach's presence in labor and delivery.
3. Attendance by Dr. X.
4. Minimal or no time in recovery room, unless maternal emergency.
5. No prep: no enema or pubic shave, unless desired.
6. Use of ice chips, juice, food, moist cloths, and pillows for comfort during labor.
7. No drugs during labor and delivery—no sedative, tranquilizer, analgesic, or anesthetic.
8. No induction of labor—unless there is risk of infection after hours of ruptured membranes with no active labor.
9. No rupture of the amniotic sac by artificial means before the baby is born.
10. No IV unless there is an emergency.
11. No use of internal or external fetal heart monitor in the absence of fetal distress; use of fetoscope for monitoring fetal heartbeat.
12. Right to assume any position desired during labor and delivery including walking, squatting, side-lying, hands and knees.
13. Lights dimmed and room quiet and warm.
14. No routine episiotomy. Use of massage to facilitate perineal stretching. If episiotomy is necessary to prevent tearing, waiting until the area is numbed by stretching and the use of xylocaine for post-episiotomy stitches rather than a pudendal block.
15. Delay cutting umbilical cord until pulsating has stopped unless cord is tight around the baby's neck or it needs immediate intensive care. Father allowed to cut the cord.
16. No silver nitrate in the eyes of the baby. Use of neosporin or other nonburning substitute delayed until one hour after the birth to allow for optimal sight for bonding.
17. Immediate exam of baby—administer APGAR scores at one and five minutes. Only remove baby from mother in case of emergency. Do newborn exam in mother's presence.
18. No removal of vernix from the baby's skin.
19. Immediate bonding—skin-to-skin contact and nursing.
20. Immediate discharge, unless there are complications, in which case rooming-in is requested.
21. No drugs administered that will dry up milk.
22. No supplemental feeding to baby (formula or sugar water).
23. Nursing on demand, both day and night.

24. No pitocin used for placental expulsion. Instead, use of nursing and nipple stimulation.
25. No cord traction or manual removal of placenta, unless there is evidence of concealed hemorrhage, bleeding before delivery of the placenta, retained placenta (past 30 minutes after the birth) or adherent placenta (past 30 minutes after the birth).
26. Massage of uterus every 15 minuts for an hour, after expulsion of the placenta.

CESAREAN DELIVERY

1. Surgery performed by OB-MD with presence of your own doctor plus the anesthesiologist you requested.
2. Presence of husband during prep, surgery and recovery.
3. Lower-segment incision (bikini cut) on uterus and abdomen, unless emergency precludes it.
4. Use of spinal anesthesia unless the baby is already severely compromised, and the speed of general anesthesia is necessary.
5. No separation of baby and parents, unless newborn emergency.
6. Immediate nursing (or as soon as possible).
7. Delay in cutting umbilical cord until it's white and not pulsating, unless baby needs immediate intensive care.
8. No silver nitrate. Use of neosporin (or other substitute) after one hour of birth to allow for optimal vision for bonding.
9. Immediate exam of baby. APGAR at one and five minutes. Father present for newborn exam and can remain with the baby.
10. No removal of vernix from baby's skin.
11. No use of supplemental feeding—demand feeding (nursing).
12. Rooming-in after recovery, unless intensive care for newborn.
13. Discharge as soon as possible.

NEWBORN COMPLICATIONS

1. Parents must be informed of baby's condition whenever requested.
2. Parents are allowed to assume as much care as possible.
3. Baby will receive colostrum or breast milk rather than formula or sugar water.
4. Nursing and rooming-in permitted as soon as possible.

A Sample Birth Plan

If the above information has not been sufficient for you, check Janet Isaacs Ashford's *Whole Birth Catalogue*[8] or *Silent Knife. Cesarean Prevention and Vaginal Birth After Cesarean* by Cohen and Estner.[9] We are including one example of a woman in childbirth classes who put together the following birth plan which was approved and supported by her doctor. Her choices may not be yours, but note the thoroughness and positive tone of her statement. Remember that you and your attendants really are on the same side, and the creation of harmony goes a long way toward getting what you want.

To My Birth Attendants:

As a parent, I have no greater concern than the health and well-being of my children. As a result, I have carefully chosen a medical team that I believe share my concern and are particularly qualified to help me make the best possible decisions in the type of health care that my children and I receive.

I accept the fact, however, that it is ultimately my responsibility to make these decisions on behalf of myself and my children, from conception through maturity. I have made every effort to gain the knowledge and information that I need to make informed decisions. It is the combination of this knowledge and careful consideration of my own values and priorities that has allowed me to determine what type of labor and delivery experience I prefer for myself and my unborn child.

I have complete faith in the normal function of the birth process. I have prepared myself through classes, prior experience, and excellent prenatal care to cope with the normal and even the more common abnormal phases of labor. I do not expect an extremely short labor or a labor without discomfort. I do expect to be allowed to labor and deliver with as few interventions as possible.

I have chosen a labor coach and a birth advocate to share my experience with me and to provide me with the emotional support I will need. I give to my birth advocate the authority to see that my preferences are carried out as closely as possible. If my physician feels that medical conditions warrant an intervention, I am willing to discuss with him the problem, the planned intervention, and its alternatives.

In order to allow my birth attendants to be able to help me achieve the type of birth experience that I wish to have, I have listed the following guidelines that are of most importance to me:

A) *That I not be separated from my coaches at any time or for any procedures unless I request it.*

B) *That I not have a perineal shave-prep.*

C) *That the amniotic membranes be allowed to rupture spontaneously.*

D) *That pelvic exams be performed only by my private physician and/or nurses.*

E) *That external fetal monitor be used only for the first 15–30 minutes after admission and then intermittently as tolerated or as medical condition warrants.*

F) *That internal fetal monitor be used only if external fetal monitor shows evidence of a problem with the infant.*

G) *That no restraints or stirrups be used at delivery and that I be allowed to deliver in a semi-sitting or side-lying position.*

H) *That episiotomy be avoided by using such methods as perineal massage and support, warm compresses, etc.*

I) *That I be allowed to drink fluids as desired throughout labor and that no glucose IV be started unless I am physically unable to take nourishment by mouth.*

J) *That delivery take place in a quiet atmosphere and that the lights be dimmed or the infant's eyes shaded at birth.*

K) *That the infant be delivered and placed directly on mother's abdomen to be observed for APGAR there.*

L) *That deep suctioning of infant be done only if suction with bulb syringe is not adequate.*

M) *That an opportunity for warm water bath be provided.*

N) *That routine newborn care be performed in the birthing/delivery room after mother has held and attempted to nurse baby, and that eye care be delayed for at least one hour.*

The following details are extremely important to me. My first child suffered from a respiratory problem during her infancy that may be hereditary. I have taken measures during my pregnancy that I hope will minimize such problems. I would like to continue this effort throughout birth through the following measures:

A) *Use of no, or absolutely minimal, medication.*
   1) *As the use of oxytocin and its derivatives may cause an increased risk of fetal distress, I ask that this not be used at all prior to birth. I also ask that the use of oxytocin immediately postpartum be delayed to allow my uterus a chance to contract naturally.*
   2) *I ask that no sedatives, analgesics, or anesthetics be given during the course of a normal labor. If, however, I decide along with my coaches that I must have something, I request that I be given nisentil, with or without benadryl.*

B) *That the umbilical cord not be clamped until it has stopped pulsating.*

C) *That no catheter be introduced into the infant to check for patency of trachea/esophagus.*

D) *That my infant absolutely not be removed from my supervision unless it requires intensive care, is under direct observation of pediatrician, or is placed on an apnea/bradycardia monitor and supervised by someone trained in its use.*

Signature _____

Date _____

◆

Dealing with Authority

If you find it extremely difficult to talk to your doctor, you can write down your questions in advance, but you might also want to explore your relationship to authority. Some of the emotion you release may help clear up your own communication cycles.

● **Review the information on women and authority in Chapter 5. What does talking to a doctor remind you of: experiences with other doctors, dentists, your father, school personnel, police?**

● **Role play a recent situation that has upset you. Try it from many different angles: as it was; if you had felt differently; if you had said what you really wanted to; if you had been the other person.**

● **Write it down: Dear Doctor** _____,
when you said _____, **I felt** _____.
**You don't realize . . . . But it's important . . . .
etc.**

- **How do you feel about your actions in such situations? Frustrated, self-righteous, idiotic? Can you accept your emotions (even tears) if they come up while talking to this authority, or do you become completely ineffectual?**

- **Think of one of the above situations, in which you got very upset. How would it have been possible to accomplish what you wanted in a more straightforward fashion? List at least five ways you could have gotten what you wanted (e.g. saying "Stop!" sooner, asking for something else, telling them something, taking someone else with you, etc.).**

_____

_____

_____

_____

_____

_____

_____

_____

_____

Questions for Midwives

It is important in considering a midwife or other homebirth attendant that communication is clear and honest and that you have a clear understanding of her training, experience, capabilities, limitations, and backup. She will also be interviewing you to see if you are informed and taking responsibility for your pregnancy and birth.

A detailed list of questions is available in *Special Delivery,* but the following areas should be covered to your satisfaction:

- Her training and experience
- How she would handle complications and emergencies
- Her assistants and medical backup

- What equipment she brings and when it would be used
- Her fee and what it covers; how prenatal care is to be arranged
- What postpartum checkups must be arranged
- What is her attitude toward birth?
- What is communication like, including:
  Does she want to be the professional in charge?
  How much responsibility does she expect, or does she "allow" you to do things?
  How involved will she be during labor, or does she primarily focus on the birth?
  How willing is she to explain things to you, to help you see the consequences of your choices, but to let you make your own choices?
  If she brings an assistant, will you get to know her as well; will they meet with your birth team?

Preparation Checklist for Homebirth

Preparation for a homebirth requires a very high level of knowledge and responsibility. *Special Delivery* was written as a complete guide for parents considering such an alternative and covers all aspects of homebirth preparation in great detail. Informed Homebirth instructor Mary Ann Copson developed the following preparation checklist for homebirth couples:

1. Have you found a skilled birth attendant with whom you feel comfortable?
2. Have you communicated to your birth attendant your desires for your pregnancy and birth?
3. Have you communicated to your birth attendant your sense of responsibility?
4. Have you read your prenatal records? Do you understand them? Do you have a copy?
5. Do you understand why certain procedures are done during your prenatal care?
6. Do you know about and understand any contra-indications and complications which might exist for you?
7. Do you know what excellent nutrition is during pregnancy? Are you eating an excellent diet?
8. Are you following an exercise program?
9. Have you met with your back-up doctor and discussed his attitudes, procedures, and treatment for emergency problems?
10. Are you familiar with the procedures of the hospital you would be using?

11. Are you informed about the complications and emergencies which may occur?
12. Have you written up your emergency back-up plan?
13. Is your birth team familiar with your emergency back-up plan?
14. Is your birth team aware of your intentions about your birth? Do they know what they will be doing?
15. Do you know what to do if your birth attendant doesn't get to the birth in time?
16. What will you do if your baby must go to the hospital?
17. Do you know where your baby will go if she needs a neonatologist?
18. Do you have a pediatrician? Do you know how he will treat certain complications? Jaundice?
19. Have you discussed your feelings about birth, death, defects, depression, quiet, if the birth does not proceed as you had planned?
20. Are you taking childbirth classes?
21. Have you contacted any other support groups? LLL, C/Sec, parenting classes?
22. Are you familiar with the normal process of labor and birth?
23. Coach—are you fully informed about labor and delivery and your partner's desires?
24. Coach—do you feel comfortable about making emergency decisions?
25. Coach—will you be able to direct the birth team?
26. Both—are you reading?
27. Are you in touch with your partner about the spiritual and psychological aspects of your birth?
28. Are your children prepared for the birth?
29. Have you gathered your birth supplies together?
30. Is your home ready for the birth?
31. How do you plan to receive your baby?
32. Are you familiar with the danger signs in a newborn?
33. Have you decided what to do about silver nitrate, circumcision, PKU test, vitamin K, jaundice?
34. Do you know how your normal post-partum recovery should proceed?
35. How do you plan to "mother the mother?"
36. Are you well-informed about breastfeeding?
37. Have you thought about and tried to plan for the immense changes in your life that a baby will bring?
38. Are you maintaining your responsibility for your pregnancy, labor, birth, baby and self?
39. Are you enjoying your pregnancy and happily anticipating the birth?

Your Husband's Role at the Birth

Most couples today want to share the birth experience. Giving birth is a unique and powerful event in a couple's relationship. For the father to be informed so he can help his wife with relaxation, massage, breathing and moral support, the couple usually attends classes together. The father is also expected to serve as patient advocate, being a calm rational voice between the medical staff and his laboring wife—this even though he is very emotionally involved with both his wife and the baby.

There is a tremendous amount to be done during labor and birth and, while we certainly advocate the sharing and support only the husband can provide, we feel it is asking a lot for him to be the only person attending the mother in labor. It is difficult for him to maintain eye-to-eye contact while he's pushing on his wife's sacrum for back labor, to give just one example. Or what about when he needs to eat or go to the bathroom? And especially as a first-time father, can he really provide the reassurance that this is normal, everything is all right, and you're doing fine?

Michel Odent speaks about women in birth responding so warmly to the midwife who quietly attends them along with their husband. He has observed that as women really enter into their bodily, instinctive selves and birth with grunts, vomiting and other physical expressions, they relate more strongly to a motherly/woman figure than to a sexual partner.[10] And in birthing where the husband has been trained as coach he sometimes spends more time watching the stop watch or fetal monitor than relating to his wife. While "coach" is a role that is easy for men to relate to, it has its limitations. Certainly Dr. Robert Bradley was right that women should share the primary emotional bonding of labor and birth with their husband, not with their obstetrician. But it is useful to think about his role at the birth.

What are you expecting from your husband? That he be there the whole time? That he is your primary support person? That he catch the baby, watch the delivery or pay attention to you at the "head end" (it's impossible to be everywhere at once!) There's no right way! The variations are as individual as we are ourselves. At Rahima's second birth, many people were present and were surrounding her with touch, so all her husband needed to do was walk around and smile. Everywhere she looked, there he was smiling, which was wonderful support. After another birth a woman was disappointed because her husband was warm and tender when she wanted him to be a pillar of rock-like support during contractions. Panuthos speaks of a birth in which the husband did nothing, the midwife was secretly furious with him, and the woman surprised them by saying to him, "Thank you, I couldn't have done it without you." Only you can communicate about what is supportive for you.

● **Discuss with your partner what is important to you during the labor and birth. How does he feel about this? What if things go differently?**

● **What's your image of how you would like to be together in labor? Joking and laughing, walking in the garden, sharing sexually?**

● **Can you act it out now to fulfill some of that desire? Your actual labor may be quite different. Even acknowledging, "This sure isn't how we thought it would be!" can help to release tension in labor and remind you of your unity.**

● **What are his feelings about his role at the birth? Does he feel that it's overwhelming? Does he feel adequately supported if at home, or does he feel that he will be able to relate positively with hospital staff?**

Very few people ever ask men about their feelings approaching labor and delivery. It's probably too scary to learn that they may feel unsure too. But it's important to share feelings to come through birth closer to each other and to the baby.

Choosing a Labor Assistant

Having a woman present who knows birth and has given birth herself can be of immeasurable support to a laboring woman, for she can provide something neither husband nor doctor can provide. Such a labor assistant can actually enhance the couple's relationship. She can be very active, or she can simply encourage and reassure you and your husband. She can also stand in for him as needed,

giving him backrubs and letting him have a few minutes off to get food or walk down the hall. You can have whatever relationship you want with a labor assistant—talk about it with your partner and with her. Sometimes your midwife or her assistant can fulfill this role, but not without discussing it with them!

If you are planning a hospital delivery, a labor assistant can be a vital help to your getting what you want. She not only encourages your husband and you during labor, but she can also be a more objective consumer advocate, helping you to weigh your own desires, the medical data and the desires of your doctor. She can remind you to ask for a second opinion, or she can be a sounding board for your own considerations should difficulties arise. She can't and shouldn't make the decisions for you, but she can be a very calming and stabilizing force during the physical and emotional involvement of labor and birth.

The comfort of having someone present who has been there herself can be of immense value in keeping up your spirits and helping you both to relax and enjoy your birth experience. Nurses unfortunately don't usually go into that kind of relationship with a birthing woman, and when shifts change, they go home and you have to try to relate to someone entirely new again. We agree with Cohen and Estner that a labor assistant is especially valuable for a woman who will be delivering vaginally after a cesarean.[11] And her presence goes a long way toward preventing unnecessary cesareans for all mothers.

While a trusted friend who is knowledgeable about birth can do very well as a labor assistant, many women seek out a childbirth educator or midwife to be their assistant. In this case, questions and services, expectations, fees, etc., should be discussed just as they would for a doctor or midwife. How available is she? Does she have a person who covers for her if she is away? Can you meet that person? Will there be enough opportunities to meet before the birth? You need to understand what is important to her and what her own birth experiences have been. What is her bias? Will she really respect you and your decisions during labor if they differ from what she would have done? Does she leave you free, but understand and support your wishes? Does she support your partner's role and the needs of your family? Is she enthusiastic, and do you feel confident around her?

Other People at the Birth

We favor the presence of a labor assistant, especially in the hospital, because it is difficult for an expectant mother and father to learn enough in a few weeks of classes to meet giving birth with all the confidence and relaxation that is possible. But we recognize that many people don't want anyone besides their husband and primary attendant present. These are choices that are yours to make. Certainly everyone's presence at a birth is keenly felt by the birthing woman, who is wide open to all the energy in the room.

In the case of hospital deliveries, where you are dealing with a string of nurses and possibly interns and students as well, it is all right to decline being used as a teaching specimen and request that your privacy be respected. If you want to be alone, nurses are usually happy to oblige when they see that you are self-assured and working well together. They have so many other women to attend to! If you are friendly and loving to one another and to the people around you, you will find that people respond in kind. They are really delighted to see a couple who know what they are doing. It is not impossible to create your own energy field in a hospital birth—you bring it with you when you come, and maintain its effectiveness with your presence.

In the case of birth center or home births where many people can be present, you need to look at your own wishes as well as those of your husband, and consider each person carefully before inviting him or her. If you invite your own mother or mother-in-law to be present, will you be relaxed and uninhibited? It can be a really wonderful experience to give birth with the woman who has given you birth, but you need to make sure your mother has an understanding of and relationship to birth similar to yours. This can be enhanced by having her read one of your books or attend classes so she knows what to expect and how to be helpful.

It is similar when considering the presence of your other children at the birth. You need to consider the power of birth and its possible effect on a young child. Children should only be present if it feels right and if they are prepared for what will happen. They need to know that blood does not mean you are hurt, and that you might make lots of noise, as you would if you were moving a piano.

And you need to feel uninhibited and supported by their presence. They also need a person who is there just for them, and who will see to their needs (labor can be long and boring for a child) and go out with them if they want to leave, even at the most crucial moment. With a young child it is sometimes better to wake them up or have them come in just after the baby comes out.

If you invite other people to be present at the birth, you might do so with the proviso that you are free to change your mind when you actually go into labor. It is difficult to know how you will really feel then, and you need to be able to make your choices without fear of hurting other people's feelings. You are the one who needs to be comfortable and have the baby. They should be there only if they are contributing, because it is possible for people to dissipate the energy at a birth and contribute to lack of progress. This is especially true if you feel that you have to perform, which we will discuss in the next chapter.

We recommend having your attendants and those who will be present meet together with you so you can discuss what is important to you, what each person can do to be most helpful, and what you want for the baby. If birthing at home, you should have a separate area where people can eat, talk, and sleep, so the energy around you remains focused.

What's Important to You for the Baby?

You and your partner need to think about what is important to you for the baby. Remembering that the baby's senses are wide open, will you want the birth to be in low light with warm temperature? If you want to do a bath such as LeBoyer described in *Birth Without Violence,* remember to have the water deep enough for the baby to be kept out of drafts. Also remember that LeBoyer was advocating attentiveness to the baby, not any set techniques or procedures.[12] If you want to do such a relaxing bath for the baby, plan to have it beside the bed so you can participate actively.

Do you have any religious practices that you want to do with the newborn, or any special ways of welcoming the baby? In many cultures the baby is presented to the earth or to the four directions or to the ancestors or the other members of the tribe.

You will also need to think about requests for the newborn as we have discussed for a hospital birth.

Or you will need to arrange in advance for a pediatrician if you are having a home birth. Issues such as circumcision, the PKU test for an enzyme deficiency, vitamin K shots, and so on, will also need to be considered (see the next chapter).

Birth Is a Doorway

Birth is something that you go *through,* into parenting. Although significant and intense, it usually lasts only a short time in comparison with the nine months of pregnancy and the decades of parenting. It is not to be focused on primarily for itself, but as a means through which your baby enters the world. Some doctors accuse women of being selfish if they talk about their requests for a hospital birth or their desire for a home delivery. Women are accused of putting their own experience and their own emotional fulfillment above the safety and well-being of their baby. This is simply not what motivates a woman, nor is it supported by the facts about safety and birth. Studies such as Lewis Mehl's and statistics from 1200 births by midwives at The Farm in Tennessee show that homebirth is not statistically less safe for the mother or baby.[13] The facts supporting birthing at home or in a birth center for women with prenatal care and a skilled attendant are too numerous to argue in this book. Suffice it to say that every woman wants what is best for her child and puts her baby above herself, whether she is birthing at home, in the hospital, having a cesarean birth or a VBAC. The values are the same, only the perceived means are different.

But there is a balance between asking for the kind of care we want, and being so annoyed by any "failures" (how we judge ourselves and others!) that we let the birth become more important than our relationship with the baby. Giving birth is an important part of a woman's life, and feelings about birth do impact parenting. But there's no such thing as the perfect birth, just as there is no such thing as a perfect year in your life if you define that as one free from disappointment, frustration or suffering. Birth is a metaphor for life. How we plan for it, how we experience it, how we feel about it afterwards are all part of who we are. All provide us with opportunities to be inwardly free and responsible as we co-create what happens to us, or to perceive ourselves as victims when things don't appear to go our way. The choices are ours.

Choices are important. They determine how you experience giving birth and how your baby enters the world. They must be made in the present and lived with in the future. If we can realize that we always make the best decision possible based on our knowledge and consciousness at the time, we can go a long way toward freeing ourselves from the past and acting with trust and faith as our life dramas unfold.

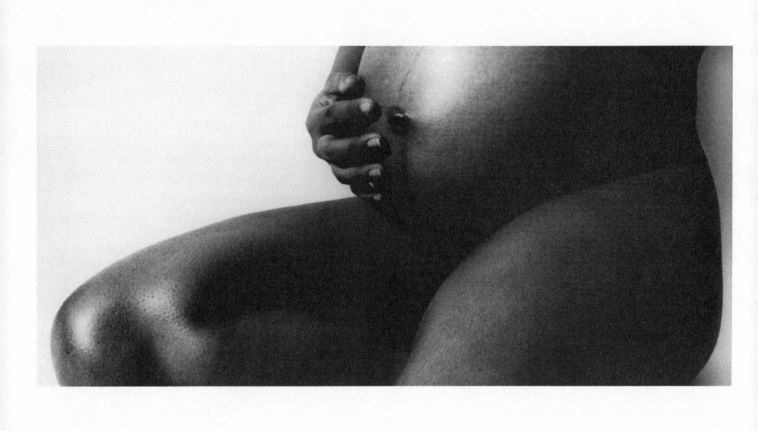

9 Opening to Birth

A woman is told she will know when she is in "real labor" because the contractions will become stronger and closer together. They develop a certain inexorable quality that builds in momentum and culminates in the birth of the baby. The similarity of birth to sexual arousal and orgasm has been noted by many writers, but Sheila Kitzinger points out that the process has perhaps erroneously been compared to the male pattern of building, building, building, explosion, instead of to the female experience of sexual arousal with its wavelike crests, valleys, and ever-higher plateaus before spilling over into orgasm. (Please note, this does not mean you will experience birth as one big orgasm or that if you are not orgasmic you will not be able to give birth!)

While most people have experienced "sex" or "sex energy," "birth energy" is not such a common idea (probably because men never experience it directly and most doctors don't sit with a woman throughout the course of labor as midwives do). Most women find that speaking of the energy present during labor and birth provides a useful image or metaphor of their experience of the increasing power of contractions during labor or its obvious lack when labor stalls or requires augmentation.

If labor is "rolling along" the best thing a woman can do during the "first stage" (dilation of the cervix) is to relax and open to its increasing intensity. Then at complete dilation everything changes: the contractions usually get further apart, and the mother feels more alert and energetic. Now she feels as if she can actively work *with* the force of contractions in pushing her baby out.

Is the power of contractions an experience of the creative power of the universe or an experience of your baby's will to be born, or simply your body's response to the physiological changes induced by your pituitary gland in response to the baby's adrenals? It doesn't matter what explanation is most satisfying to you, you can still recognize that your own energy and your experience of contractions will be different at two centimeters dilation than at nine centimeters. While progress is most often checked by internal exams, an experienced midwife can follow the course of labor by monitoring the energy present. She reads cues from the woman's skin tone, her eyes, her talkativeness, the hardness of her belly during contractions, and whether her focus is external or internal.

This chapter discusses the changes in energy during the labor and delivery and how it is possible to work in harmony with that energy in giving birth to your baby. After discussing normal labor and delivery, we look at ways of releasing the energy when it is blocked (often called "uterine inertia," or "failure to progress"). By understanding how to work with energy as birthing women and attendants, we can help to avoid these problems in the first place.

In Early Labor
As Labor Begins

How, in fact, does labor start? Scientists have demonstrated that there is a complex interaction of chemical harmones, some of which are initiated by the baby itself. So it seems the baby has a say in determining the exact moment of birth. Certainly labor should be allowed to start naturally whenever a nonemergency cesarean is being done, to assure both the maturity of the baby and a more natural time of birth. It is another sign of our desire for control that elective cesareans are done at the physician's convenience rather than when the baby is ready to be born.

Why does labor most often start in the middle of the night? Probably because a woman is more relaxed then, and most open to the energy of birth. Nurses on maturity wards will tell that they are most crowded around the full moon. Is there really such a connection? We haven't seen any scientific studies to document it, but we wouldn't be surprised!

How will you know you are in labor? Contractions become stronger and closer together. Some women have pre-labor contractions—opportunities during the last months of pregnancy to practice their breathing and relaxation with contractions that go away after a few minutes or a few hours. This is quite normal and is a good sign that your body is warming up for the task. We don't need to call these "Braxton-Hicks contractions" after two men who "discovered them," nor are they "false labor" (in the sense of being something negative or unreal).

Before going into labor, you may experience the nesting urge, or a natural loosening of your bowels, or the release of the mucus plug which has been in the opening of the uterus (it can be pink or dark brown and is stringy like egg white). These are all signs that birth is approaching. The loss of the mucus plug is a very positive sign that your uterus is ripening and starting to open in preparation for labor. You will probably go into labor within the next few days. If your waters break, which only happens before labor in 10 percent of pregnancies, get your things together and then sit back and relax, because you will soon be going into labor (almost always within 24 hours).

The Excitement of Early Labor

During early labor, the best thing you can do if it is night is to go back to sleep. Even though it's exciting, you don't know how long labor will last. Your body may kick in and you can have the baby in a few hours, or you may have two days of this kind of early labor and then go into active labor. Don't waste your resources on early labor—if you can rest or sleep, do so. We can guarantee you won't sleep through the birth!

Early labor can be very exciting: It is really happening, where is everyone, do we have everything ready, is it snowing? A dozen questions race through your mind. Such considerations can lead to physical tension that makes you wonder, "How will I ever get through active labor if it hurts this much now?" Relaxing, taking a warm bath, sleeping, or getting a massage can help to smooth your nerves and your muscles. You can become more comfortable with early labor, and you do have the resources to deal with later labor.

During early labor, a woman is often excited and outgoing. It's really best not to think of yourself as being in labor and not to notify anyone except your primary attendant. If you are birthing in the hospital, don't go until you have really reached the criteria your doctor has set, especially with first births. If you don't consider yourself in labor until you have reached 4 centimeters, you won't have such a long labor, you'll have more energy, and you won't be discouraged by the fact that it usually takes much longer to go from 2 to 3 centimeters than from 7 to 8 centimeters. Understanding early labor can really help women stay focused and not get discouraged if they have a long *latent phase,* as it is called. Rest, walk around, cook, knit, read. If you aren't sleeping, stay vertical and active, breathing with contractions only as you need to.

Early labor is a wonderful time to hug and kiss with your partner. It's an exciting time—a time of anticipation and a time to be close, your last opportunity to be together without a new baby. And it is your last chance to experience your pregnant body. Say goodbye to being pregnant, and remember that birth is just a doorway you are going *through* to being as successful a mother to this child on the outside as you have been while he or she was on the inside. Welcome the energy of birth, welcome the increasing intensity of the contractions that will bring your baby closer to you. Share this energy with your partner, let it flow to him during a contraction. If you feel like hugging and kissing, do so! The Farm midwives pointed out that the same energy that got your baby in will help get your baby out.[1] Stay released, stay loose. Nipple stimulation will produce natural oxytocin, which stimulates contractions. This is especially true if it feels good! Have your partner roll your nipples between his fingers as he caresses and loves you; tell him what feels good. Open to the energy that is birthing your baby.

Think of images of opening. Imagine your cervix opening over your baby's head. Or envision a flower opening. What other images come to you? Focus, too, on the baby. Something to help you do that during labor is the following baby-uterus exercises, which you can do now with your partner or a friend.

Baby-Uterus Exercise

You will be the baby and your partner will be the uterus for this exercise. Then when it is finished, trade roles without talking. Once you have both had the chance to experience being the baby, then discuss what you felt. Here's how to do it:

1. Read these directions first, so you can do it without them.

2. Choose a room with a comfortable rug or mats and make the lighting soft. Take off your shoes and glasses. Make sure you have time and no interruptions.

3. The person who is to be the baby first lies on her side, curled tightly into the fetal position.

4. The person who is to be the "uterus" lies along the length of his partner's body, with hands clasped in a circle over the top of her head. He should put his weight on her hip bones, in order not to squash the real baby.

5. Now that you're in position, please maintain silence and a serious mood for the exercise to be effective. The uterus will contract, becoming heavier and tighter around the baby. Hold . . . . and then release. Pause a while and then do another contraction. Take your time.

6. Keep up a slow rhythm of contractions, gradually letting them become stronger. At some point the baby can start moving her head, as if trying to get out. But the uterus holds firm. The circle of fingers on her head widens gradually, and during one contraction, his hands open over her head and rest on her neck during the next pause. The head has been born.

7. During the next, final contraction, slide the hands all the way down her body until you get to the feet as the baby is born!

8. Maintain silence while she experiences being a newborn. When she is ready, trade roles. She assumes the position of the uterus and he becomes the baby. Repeat the exercise.

9. Once you have both experienced the birth, share together what it was like being the baby. What was your experience when you were inside? What were contractions like? Was it hard to breathe? (Remember, your baby has the umbilical cord, but there is some compression and lessening of oxygen during each contraction.) What did you feel as soon as you were out? What did you want?

The above exercise can give you a real insight into what it is like for the baby during labor. It can give you a kind of body knowledge or memory of birth, because unless you were born by cesarean section, you and your partner both had that experience. After this exercise, focusing on the baby during labor can go beyond an abstract thought. You may be able to tune into the baby inside you in a way that isn't possible with the mind alone.

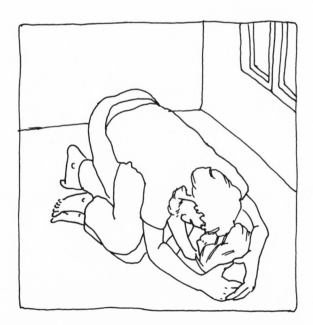

Various Women's Dialogues with Birthing Energy (B.E.)

B.E.: I'm here.

Me: Welcome. But, what if I want you to go away? I'm scared.

B.E.: Go with me and you needn't fear.

Me: OK. I'll trust my body to you.

B.E.: Here we go!

B.E.: I'm ready to be with you. It's time to deliver the baby.

Me: I'm ready, and I'm feeling happy to become a mother.

B.E.: I'll be coming stronger and stronger and I'm here to assist you.

Me: I get that I need you.

B.E.: If you'll ride me like a wave you won't go under, you'll just get higher.

Me: That sounds great. What if I feel like you're too much for me?

B.E.: If you feel that, just be with it. I'll never be more than you can handle. You can handle it.

Me: I need that reassurance now and then.

B.E.: You've got it; you're as powerful as I am when we unite and work together.

Me: Great.

B.E.: Connect with someone else and share my energy when it feels like too much for you to handle alone. Share my energy and let it flow. There's exactly the amount that's needed to do our task of delivering this baby into the world.

Me: I'm feeling more assured now that we can do it together.

B.E.: Let's go! Let's be!

Me: Hello.

B.E.: Hi. Are you ready for me?

Me: No! Wait a minute.

B.E.: I can't wait. Here I am. Experience me.

Me: OK. OK. (deep breaths)

B.E.: See, that wasn't so bad.

Me: Hey—no it wasn't. Having a baby isn't so painful after all.

B.E.: Oh, yeah? Here I come again.

Me: (deep breaths) Hey! Why did you have to get more intense?

B.E.: That's the game, baby.

Me: OK. Well, I'm still going to relax and enjoy this. Joanna and Andrew, would you please play some soothing music?

B.E.: Here I come again.

Me: That's OK. You don't scare me. (deep breaths) I've got lots of love and support and breathing techniques and, most of all, faith in the Lord. "Thou wilt keep him in perfect peace whose mind is stayed on Thee because he trusteth in Thee." (Isaiah 26:3)

Me: What do you do during labor?

B.E.: I move through you.

Me: What do you want me to do?

B.E.: Welcome me.

Me: You're not scary to me now, but you were the first time.

B.E.: You resisted.

Me: I know. I wasn't ready yet.

Me: So, now we've met, and I'd like to work with you.

B.E.: Good.

Me: I want to open.

B.E.: Good.

Me: Let's be one together and flow with the combining of our energies.

B.E.: Good. As each contraction begins, a deep cleansing breath will help in centering this flow. As you breathe, visualize energy traveling down through yourself and out your birth canal. This energy will be traveling in a circle. Inhale love and light into your belly. Then exhale out the birth canal, feeling the baby moving down.

Me: Let's begin. I feel your presence strongly.

In Active Labor

One of the beautiful things about labor is that it happens over time, allowing your body to adapt to the increasing intensity. Many people hope for a short labor, but short labors are often very intense or can leave a woman in shock that she has the baby so soon.

How long does labor last? What can we answer except, "Until the baby is born." Whether your labor is long or short, one of the most important things is to *stay in the present moment*. Women who are having short labors, or who have progressed further than they have been told they should expect, often look ahead and feel, "I can't go on like this for hours longer!" And they're right, for the baby is only twenty minutes away. Better to feel it and be with it and know that you won't be given more than you can bear. And if a labor is long, thinking of how long it has been or how long you think you have to go can be discouraging. Rather, stay with what is, breathing, relaxing and opening. The baby will come out.

"Progress" is a similar snare that can catch us and take us out of the present moment. Remember that each contraction brings you closer to holding your baby in your arms. In *Spiritual Midwifery*, Ina May Gaskin offered the wonderful advice, "Think about the opening, not the contracting."[2] Although dilation usually becomes more rapid as contractions increase in intensity, labor is not a textbook curve as it is taught in medical school. There can be pauses, plateaus, times when your body is resting or the baby is turning. Often at full dilation there is a pause before the pushing urge establishes itself. If your baby's heart tones remain good and you are not exhausted, there is no reason for alarm—labor can change at any moment, and the baby will come out.

A woman in active labor is often more inward, more concentrated on the work that she is doing. Sometimes the things that felt good at an earlier stage no longer feel good, so keep in good communication with your attendants. Ask for what you need, and express your appreciation. If you feel like talking, try saying what you are doing to help you focus on it. "I'm opening." "I love you baby." Channelling love to your baby, your husband and your attendants can help the energy flow through you rather than become blocked.

Sound can help energy flow through you. If you want to be vocal, don't be afraid what people will think. Try making sounds during a contraction that will help with opening. These would be *oh* or *ah* sounds, which are deep and rounded, as opposed to *eee* sounds that come from high in the body through a closed throat. Because of the neurological connection between your throat and vagina, a closed throat also indicates tension in your pelvic floor. Let it all go. Let out a war whoop or a tremendous grunt if you want to. Release any tension. Then focus again on your breathing during contractions.

You can't control labor, but you can control yourself. Control in this sense means the freedom to decide how to respond in a situation, rather than behaving in a certain way. Whether you go through a contraction smiling beatifically, or breathing, or grunting and bellowing like the Earth Mother, is only a question of style if *you* are deciding rather than being at the mercy of labor or "out of control" (i.e. feeling victimized). You don't need to *behave* in labor; you especially don't need to "behave like a lady." But you can decide to be positive, or to relax, or to make sounds, or to swear. The choices are yours. Birth is really a microcosm for all of life. We can't control other people or the weather or what happens to us, but we do have the possibility to choose how we interpret and respond to all of those situations. If we can have confidence in ourselves and the tools we have for dealing with the intensity of labor, then we can realize our freedom to birth with joy and exhilaration, rather than conforming to anything imposed from the outside.

Elizabeth Nobel, in *Childbirth with Insight*, describes it very well: "Birthing with insight, a mother freely finds her own labor positions, makes sounds without inhibition, enjoys support and caresses from her partner and chosen attendants, eats to appetite, drinks to thirst, and generally responds in a way that feels natural for her. In a liberal birth environment, such as an alternative birth center or at home, she does not have to worry about how her behavior is viewed by others or whether she is conforming to a certain method of birth.[3]"

In going beyond techniques, it is necessary to affirm a woman's own power and ability to birth. She needs to reclaim the center of focus of the birthing process. Attendants need to take their cues from her, serving her, safeguarding her, and allowing her to experience her unique labor and delivery, rather than trying to get her to conform to standards of performance which serve their own ideas, convenience or comfort.

Anything that really serves the mother encourages the birthing energy during active labor. Those things that encourage lovemaking also further birth: low lighting, low noise, few distractions, loving touch, encouraging words. All of these can help a laboring woman, but her attendants have to be receptive to her, and to her changes. If she becomes less verbal, she may push a hand away. What felt good in early labor may not feel good now.

Women should eat and drink during labor. In hospitals we are told not to, "just in case you need a cesarean," but we need energy, energy from food, not glucose water. Food is digested during labor, and if it is thrown up (which sometimes happens), the muscular release from vomiting will help to open the cervix and pelvic-floor muscles. Blender drinks, soups, juice made into ice chips, pizza, whatever you want should be available. You should also be free to walk around, since walking and squatting increase the strength of contractions, bringing the baby's head down while opening the pelvis and decreasing the time of labor.

The Moment of Surrender

There often comes a time of tension in late labor, just before full dilation of the cervix. Think about putting a t-shirt on your head—or better yet, on a toddler's head. The opening enlarges, getting bigger and bigger until there is a point of maximum tension, just before the head goes through. If you feel the sides of your own head, you will understand why that tension occurs. Those ridges are called the bi-parietal bosses. When your uterus is at that point of maximum tension and stretch before your baby's head starts to descend down the birth canal, you may not know whether you are coming or going. You may feel hot and cold at the same time, and contractions may be back-to-back. Was that a contraction with three peaks or three contractions? The reason for this is that both your sympathetic and parasympathetic nervous system are being stimulated at the same time when your uterus is nearly completely open. It can be fairly chaotic, like being adrift in a stormy sea. Keep yourself anchored in your partner's eyes, or in thinking about the baby, or in positive statements, and in the knowledge that this will soon pass into the release of full dilation and the descent of the head.

This time of tension was dramatically demonstrated to Rahima when she was at a birth with midwife Jesusita Aragon, who at the time was 74 years old and had attended more than 15,000 births. At one point in the woman's labor, Jesusita started to yawn and yawn. Rahima, feeling fairly useless anyway and wanting to be helpful, asked Jesusita if she was tired and if there was anything she needed. "Oh no," was her reply. "I always yawn when they are in transition." Sure enough, shortly thereafter the head started to be visible. Without checking dilation, Jesusita knew where the woman was simply by the energy in the room. (Yawning is a common response to a certain kind of "sticky" energy.)

This time of greatest intensity can bring up natural doubts like "Can I do it? or "Can I go on?" Everyone present also goes through their own

doubts, like "What if something goes wrong?" or "Why am I a midwife?" Recognize them as a welcome sign that everything will soon release.

At the moment when the energy seems as if it is too powerful, there is a surrender and a tremendous release of tension. As midwives we have seen this surrender occur quite naturally and unconsciously with most women. It is similar to the surrender necessary to have an orgasm—you can't hang on, and you can't control it, and you can't keep it all together or you won't have one. The energy sweeps through you and over you like a wave, and you come out on the other side. We have also helped women who have had long or stalled labors consciously come to that point of deciding to surrender rather than hold the energy at bay or feel discouraged or like a failure. The result has been a tremendous burst of power and the birth of the baby. There's no way around it except forceps or cesarean. You have to open, and you will be all right.

In Birth

The "other side" that most women come out on is usually what is called *second stage*. This is where the cervix is completely open and the baby is coming down the birth canal, and then starting to be visible at the vaginal opening. The vagina, full of accordian folds, opens easily. The baby crowns and is born. How long this takes depends on many factors, including the size of the baby and the position of its head. With women who have already had children, this can take only a few contractions, as the release of full dilation and the birth of the baby merge.

With first-time mothers, however, second stage can often last two hours or longer. But the change in the energy is dramatic. Once a husband at a birth went out when the mother was dilated about 8 centimeters. She appeared exhausted and spacy, was working very hard and did not relate much to those around her. When he returned she was actively pushing, and he couldn't believe the difference. She was sitting up, bright-eyed, vibrant, and tremendously excited. Contractions were further apart and felt very different to her. She was actively able to work with them in birthing her baby, and the energy had totally changed. Following the complete opening of the cervix, the baby actually starts to move and the energy of labor gives way to the work and excitement of birth.

Rather than acting like cheerleaders and exhorting

women to "PUSH!" while the coach yells from the sidelines and the doctor prepares to catch the baby like a football, we encourage women to continue breathing through contractions, feeling what each one is doing and saying to her. Contractions in second stage are usually further apart than at the height of labor, and it is possible actually to feel the baby's head descending in the vagina. We tend to think of the birth canal as being 500 miles long; the 3 to 4 inches the baby travels are a short but remarkable journey!

Women who continue breathing with contractions either feel the baby start to come down, in which case they can probably breathe the baby right out, or they feel a pushing urge grow in strength. First felt as a catch in the throat, the urge to push can begin any time in active labor or second stage, or it may not manifest at all. Caused by pressure of the baby's head against the rectum, it feels similar to needing to have a bowel movement and starts as an involuntary catch in the throat. Women are sometimes told to "resist the pushing urge" until they are fully dilated. This is impossible; you can no more resist an involuntary pushing urge than you can resist your heartbeat. What is meant is not to go into "full pushing mode" before the cervix is completely over the baby's head or it can become swollen and impede progress. What you should do instead is breathe through the pushing urge just as you have breathed through contractions, until it becomes so overwhelming that there's nothing else to be done.

Many women are able to breathe their baby out with no more effort than having a bowel movement if they aren't exhorted to push.[4] The fact that this possibility exists, combined with studies by Caldeyro Barcia and others showing that holding the breath for longer than 6 or 7 seconds can compromise the baby, has lead many childbirth educators and women to advocate "responsive pushing," rather than the athletic model so often demanded. When this is done, Sheila Kitzinger suggests that the energy of second stage comes in waves, much as women experience sexual energy in making love. The male model of tension, tension, tension, explosion, which has been used until now is not one that fits the female body or feminine images.

While some women breathe their babies out, others need to push quite hard for a long time. In fact, they are astounded by the force of the energy birthing their baby. There is no set technique for pushing, just as there is none for lovemaking. But imitating the stirrups position by lying down and holding your legs in the air must be second only to being hung by your heels as far as being unphysiologically sound. If you're confined to a delivery table, there's nowhere to put your legs, but if you're in a bed, let them fall open or simply squat. If you or your attendants are concerned about second stage or getting the baby out, assume a supported squatting position with someone holding you under the arms. Such a supported squat is a common birthing position at Odent's clinic in Pithiviers. This supported position suspends a woman without effort while she is working with gravity. Squatting with your arm around someone next to you also works with gravity and helps to open the pelvis. Not only do contractions become stronger and more effective, but the baby has a clearer pathway out instead of having to go uphill around the pubic bone.

Many midwives encourage women to squat during labor or second stage, but would have them lie back for perineal support for the birth of the head. Films such as "Birth in the Squatting Position" from a metropolitan clinic in Brazil show women squatting and popping out their babies without any perineal support.[5] Pressure is supposedly equalized by being in an upright squat, so there is no need to support the perineum from tearing. The rate of tears is said to be as low or lower than in other positions, but solid data was unavailable to us at this time.

If you do not decide to squat for the birth of the head, you will probably want to have a doctor or midwife doing perineal support and using oil or hot compresses. The ineffective method of pushing with tremendous effort until the crowning, then stopping and blowing for the final contraction, always reminded us of those cartoons in which the character runs off the edge of the cliff while trying to stop. It is nearly impossible to stop and blow when the head actually comes out if you've been forcefully pushing until then. Having a much more gentle, responsive second stage can enable a woman to work with her body and her attendants to birth her baby's head without undue force or tearing of the tissues of the vagina or perineum.

When your baby's head is showing, reaching down and touching it reminds you what you are working for and can be a tremendous help in keeping your energy up during second stage. The head is so inner and yet so other! If you want to touch your baby, it is your right to do so, and you needn't worry about causing infection.

With the birth of the head there is a tremendous release of pressure, and then often a timeless pause before the rest of the body is born. Your baby may shoot out, or there may be as much as three minutes before the next contraction births the shoulders—minutes which can seem like an eternity. Your baby is literally between two worlds, no longer a fetus and not yet a newborn.

The shoulders and body usually come out without difficulty on the next contraction. Bringing your baby up to your belly is something you are free to do. You don't need anyone to deliver the baby or to hand it to you. *You* have done this work. The work of Drs. Moyses and Claudio Paciornick with city women in Brazil birthing in the squatting position is interesting because they don't just scoop the baby up. The women are very tentative in looking at and touching the baby for a few moments and are allowed this time to touch and then hold the baby without being interrupted.[6] A watchful eye by the attendant is usually all that is necessary. In an upright position, the mother is self-sufficient and able to relate to a slippery baby without fear of its falling off the table.

Right After the Birth

As your baby comes out, remember to keep breathing. He or she is still getting some oxygen from the placenta and will start to breathe and pink up within a minute. As your baby makes faces, starts to make sounds and takes the first breath of earthly life, the elation you will feel is indescribable. Everyone may have to make a real effort to maintain quiet if that is what you want for the baby. The sense of release and achievement and awe are extremely powerful. They are often missed in a hospital setting where the woman has had a spinal anesthesia and the baby is whisked off to an isolette while the doctor begins to repair her episiotomy.

Pitocin is often given in the hospital to deliver the placenta while it is pulled out with cord traction within the first three minutes. But placentas really do come out naturally, and are wonderful because they have no bones! Squatting is also the ideal position in which to birth the placenta because of the effect of gravity. In the excitement of having a new baby, don't forget that the birth is not completed until you deliver the placenta and your uterus clamps down. When you feel a contraction, midwives will usually have you squat over a bowl for the placenta, which comes away and is delivered within about twenty minutes.

In the time following the birth, allow your attendants to watch the baby and monitor your bleeding.

Just relax and enjoy being with your baby and your partner. Uninterrupted time together is really valuable here. The baby is usually awake and alert during the first 30 to 60 minutes following the birth, and it is a good time to start to get to know one another on the outside.

What About Bonding?

Marshall Klaus, who together with John Kennel did some of the most visible work on the importance of parent-infant bonding, says there is no critical time for bonding in humans as there is in some animals. Bonding for us is the process of an adult's forming an attachment to a baby, making the space in his or her life for loving and caring for this other being (24 hours a day, whether or not you are tired, etc.). Children don't need to bond with their parents. It happens naturally, since babies *are* love, and children will even love parents who mistreat them.

As busy adults, however, we need to bond with our children, and studies have been done in which bonding failed to occur because of lack of contact with a sick or premature newborn. There was shown to be a marked correlation between a lack of bonding and cases of child abuse and socially aberrant behavior when the child grew up. Similarly, Klaus's further studies showed that *any* increased time of mother-infant contact resulted in "better parenting" according to their behavior scales.

Bonding, however, is something that goes on throughout pregnancy, continues through the birth and into an infant's life. In a follow-up study by Klaus, 97 mothers were asked when they first felt love for their babies. Forty-one percent replied during pregnancy; twenty-four percent at the birth; twenty-seven percent during the first week; and eight percent after the first week. Bonding is an ongoing process. It doesn't happen once and forever, nor is it missed once and forever. We see bonding as a present-time phenomenon, something that occurs any time you treat another person as a human being instead of an object.

We have brought up these points because so many women feel guilty if they have been separated from their babies for the first half-hour due to cesarean anesthesia, having to be stitched, or for whatever reason. If birth is a tremendous letdown— if you work so hard, only to have a spinal at the end, and then the baby is whisked away—you can feel discouraged or depressed. *This* influences bonding, not the fact that you weren't holding your baby during the first twenty minutes. Mothers and babies belong together, without any unnecessary separation. Hospitals need to recognize this and have newborn exams done in the mother's presence. It is more important to change those procedures than to have "bonding rooms" that only give lip service to the concept.

There is similarly no critical time with breast-feeding. Your baby begins sucking in utero. In fact, some babies are born with calluses on their thumbs from sucking so much. So your baby will probably want to suck when he or she is born. But there isn't a critical time that you have to catch or lose it. Sucking at the breasts helps the baby get used to nursing and stimulates the mother's uterus to expel the placenta and then stop bleeding. Bottles, which release their contents so much more easily, should be avoided. With no separation, there will not be theoretical questions such as, "Should the baby nurse on the delivery table?" Parents and attendants can be sensitive to the energy of the birth and the energy this baby brings with it!

If you try to tune into your baby, you will become aware of what he or she wants. Perhaps it is to be held, perhaps to nurse, perhaps to be placed in a tub of warm water. Attention to the baby all during labor and delivery and especially once he or she is born is of tremendous importance. Babies' senses are wide open to light, temperature, sounds and touch. There aren't any formulas, and the baby shouldn't have to be sacrificed to institutional procedures. Many things done routinely are unnecessary, including suctioning with a bulb syringe. It's important to have one available, but it's possible to see if the baby breathes and whether or not the mucus comes out by itself. Babies don't need to be scrubbed—the vernix is good for the skin and can be rubbed in. They should be checked by a midwife or pediatrician, but it can be done while the mother holds the baby!

Various Women's Dialogues with Birthing Energy (B.E.)

Me: What's up?
B.E.: It's happening. Just stay relaxed. It'll be okay.
Me: And all my apprehensions, hopes?
B.E.: They're okay too. Lot's of emotion, peace. This is the time to pour them out along with everything else. Trust yourself. Trust your body. Trust Zeke. Trust your friends.
Me: Help me through.

B.E.: We all will.
Me: Thank you.

◆

Me: You're so strong.
B.E.: So are you.
Me: Are you stronger than me?
B.E.: Is the liquid stronger than the bottle?
Me: I'm bursting. I can't hold it.
B.E.: Let go, let go.
Open, let it flow.
Me: Uuuuuh.
B.E.: Mmmmmh.
Me: I'm so strong now.
B.E.: We both are.
Me: We're a team.
B.E.: We are one.
Me: You are a wave.
B.E.: You are the ocean.
Me: Come on.
B.E.: Let go.
Me: Love. Open. O-o-pen!
B.E.: Love.
Me: Come . . .
B.E.: Go.

◆

Me: Greetings, dear energy. You are going to help me see my baby.
B.E.: You must stay with me.
Me: Where are we going?
B.E.: Nowhere, everywhere with the energy, in the energy, up, out and through.
Me: Can I do it? Will we be together?
B.E.: If you let it go. Don't try. Nothing is more than you can stand.
Me: Will you tell me what to do?
B.E.: You will know if you let go.
Me: I want to feel the infinite connection.
B.E.: It's there, here.
Me: Help me feel it, share it!

◆

B.E.: Hi!
Me: I can't look you in the eye. I feel like you could take me away.
B.E.: You can resist me or you can invite me, but I am coming. I will be birthing your baby one way or the other—with your consent or without it. Invite me to be with you. After all, I'm bringing your beautiful baby.

◆

B.E.: I am strong and I will do what is necessary to bring the baby into the world. Relax and work with me. Relax *and allow me to work. This energy is the same energy that flowed through your mother and gave birth to you.*

The energy prepares the baby for entrance into the world. It has been nine months of warmth, darkness and stillness. Now the baby is about to enter a world of light, sound and air. The birth is a transition between these two worlds. The contractions massage and propel.

Me: *I am ending one phase and beginning another life.*

B.E.: *I will guide you through the transition.*

Me: *Having a baby, another human being doesn't seem real.*

B.E.: *I will make this real for you.*

Me: *Are you gliding in tonight to stay?*

B.E.: *I've come to glide through you. We'll glide together into motherhood.*

Me: *I must prepare myself.*

B.E.: *Be calm, you are prepared.*

Me: *Where should I begin—in the bedroom . . .*

B.E.: *Begin inside yourself. We begin our practice now with a gentle contraction— rising, rising.*

Me: (little voice) *I'm frightened . . .*

B.E.: *There's no need, see how easily we've glided through this one.*

Me: *The poor baby . . .*

B.E.: *The baby will be fine. It is excited and ready to glide down.*

Me: *We will glide through this together. My baby and I will be the birthing energy.*

B.E.: *Here we go.*

Me: *Oh, so good to see you! Will you be here long?*

B.E.: *As long as it takes. Hang in there.*

Me: *Will it hurt?*

B.E.: *That's in large part up to you. Are you afraid?*

Me: *A little . . .*

B.E.: *You are one of countless women who have/are/will give birth. You have the strength if you trust and respect it. Your body is a miracle. Respect it and enjoy our time together!*

Me: *Okay. It's getting intense.*

B.E.: *You are part of the flow. Go with it.*

Me: *Okay.*

B.E.: *Be here now. Just this rush. Can you handle just this rush?*

Me: *Yeah.*

B.E.: *Good.*

Me: *It feels like a freight train going through me.*

B.E.: *You're doing so well! Ride with the train.*

Me: *I don't know how long I can do this.*

B.E.: *Think about your baby instead of the rush.*

Me: *Come home, Baby. Come out so I can kiss you.*

B.E.: *The time is* now.

Me: *Oh, thanks, I've been so anxiously waiting.*

B.E.: *I'll get stronger and stronger.*

Me: *Oh, please, be strong enough to make the baby come quickly. Why does it take so long?*

B.E.: *Slow and sure wins the race.*

Me: *This bulge is so intense! Why don't we become numb to the* intense *numbness?*

B.E.: *So you can carry these treasured memories.*

Me: *Why do you make me uptight with my husband whom I love most?*

B.E.: *That is* my *secret.*

Me: *Thanks so for the confidence I have in myself.*

B.E.: *You give more than you thought was possible.*

Me: *I know, and I get even more. Thanks for the memories.*

Releasing Blocks
When the Energy is Blocked Going into Labor

As you contemplate going into labor, remember that only 5 percent of women deliver on their due date. Two hundred and eighty days is an average that is helpful to your attendant, but doesn't say how long *your* baby will need to be on the inside before coming out. It can be annoying to go past your due date. Friends and relatives often call and seem to be saying, "Are you still around? Hasn't anything happened yet?" Remember to trust that the baby will be born in his or her own perfect time. And relax. Surrender. You can't determine when it will begin. But if you are really overdue, you can help release any blocks to the energy by trying chiropractic adjustment, lovemaking, acupuncture massage, or two tablespoons of castor oil mixed with a little orange juice. Castor oil gives you the runs, and the peristalsis of the bowels can get your uterus going *if* it is ripe and ready to go into labor. Otherwise, you'll just have a good cleansing! Be sure to let your birth attendant know any decision about starting labor.

You can also look at your life situation and any fears that you may have about giving birth or being a mother. Just that looking, acknowledging and letting go can be enough to allow labor to start. Sometimes your baby just needs to "cook" longer. But other times it is possible to keep labor at bay. A mother animal, for example, will not go into labor or will completely stop labor if she does not feel safe. In the same way, a woman whose husband is ill, who must work until her due date, or who must move her home can be late going into labor until her life settles and she feels able to give birth in peace. A woman who is in labor can also experience a temporary stopping of contractions when she goes through all the flurry of hospital admission or of changing from labor to delivery room. Dilation can even decrease; the uterus can shut down due to the complex interaction of mind and body.

As you near your due date, prepare those things you need to have ready, and relax. The nesting urge is well-known and can be a positive sign, but resist washing all the drapes in the house, tearing up the kitchen floor, and becoming exhausted. It's important to be well-rested when you go into labor!

If you go past your due date, you may encounter concern from your doctor. The major danger in postmaturity (defined as three or more weeks past a known due date) is that the placenta, which has its own life cycle, can start to decrease in efficiency and the baby may not be receiving enough nourishment. Postmature babies can have large, more calcified heads with thin bodies if the placenta has not been providing adequate nourishment. If your placenta is healthy (no bleeding), you don't smoke (which can cause calcified spots on the placenta), and your nutrition has been excellent (high protein, salt and fluids to taste), then your baby is probably in fine form. If your attendant is overly concerned, you should first check your due dates by noting any irregularities in your periods or possible miscalculation of the time of conception. Gestational size throughout pregnancy can also give clues to gestational age. Noninvasive tests that can be done to reassure the doctor of placental sufficiency include an estriol check, in which your urine is checked twice within twenty-four hours to see if the level is steady and not declining (estriol is a by-product of placental function). If it is good, you don't need any further tests.

The next level of testing is the Non-Stress Test, in which the mother is hooked up to a fetal monitor and blood-pressure cuff and she says every time she feels the baby move. The technician wants to see so much movement in a given period of time and so much variation in heart tones each time the baby moves. The stressful part of this "non-stress test" is going into the testing environment and having to perform (which can change your blood pressure) and getting inconclusive results, which is often the case. Different hospitals have different criteria for passing the test, and there is a wide range of gray area which *shouldn't* make you feel more uncertain than before, but it usually does.

The next level of testing is the Stress Test, which measures how your baby, whom they fear might be compromised, responds to contractions induced by pitocin, which are stressful. Going in for a stress test is dangerously close to getting a cesarean, because if you don't have adequate contractions you have failed to be induced into labor; and if you do have adequate contractions, your baby may not like them. A cesarean can be recommended in either case.

If you find yourself several weeks late, work with yourself, your attendants and your partner, and go into labor without requiring all these agonies. Sometimes it really is a question of giving up, or letting go. Talk to the baby and tell him or her what's happening, what you feel, and what is needed. Either go into labor, or you will have to make your own decisions about the risks and the tests.

Uncertainty and anxiety can also creep in if your waters break and you don't go into labor right away. Counteract them with the knowledge and certainty that it is time for your baby to be born, your body is ripe and ready, and labor will begin. When the waters break, it is almost always followed by labor within 24 hours. The best thing you can do is get your things together, and then relax. *Don't* call everyone or don't go to the hospital right away. Go back to sleep if it is night, or enjoy the time with your partner if he is home during the day. Hug, kiss, stimulate your nipples and clitoris, and enjoy yourselves, but intercourse and vaginal exams are contraindicated because you and the baby are open to infection.

There is concern among many doctors that the baby be delivered within 24 hours due to the risk of infection. Other doctors are more willing to wait, monitoring the mother's temperature and sometimes prescribing antibiotics prophylactically. However, studies by Kloosterman et al have shown that the risk of infection with broken waters does not increase after 24 hours if vaginal exams are not done.[7] So relax, let go of being pregnant, and surrender to the energy of birth that is about to be with you. Walking, showering (water stimulation of the nipples) and emotional openness all keep the energy from becoming blocked.

Being a Performer

Nan's Class, a film shown by many childbirth educators, starts out with a woman whose waters break. She is excited and dutifully calls her doctor and goes to the hospital. We watch as she sits in the labor room, with nothing but her husband and a huge clock on the wall. Every few hours a nurse or the doctor comes in and asks, "Nothing happening yet?" Her smiles slowly change to concern and finally to discouragement. The clock ticks away, the ax falls, and she has a cesarean section. In the meantime we're sitting in the auditorium, silently screaming and yelling and jumping out of our seats—another unnecessary cesarean caused by counterproductive instructions and anxiety. With that kind of pressure to "perform" and without any attention to what would help labor get started, she didn't have a chance.

This woman, like so many others, was caught by insensitivity to what furthers birth. Pressure to perform hinders birth just as it does getting an erection. In the hospital, pressure can come from the necessity to conform to Friedman's curve of so many centimeters per hour of dilation. Or you can feel like an idiot at home if you've called all your friends over from work when your waters break, but then there's no labor. Standards from the outside and our own expectations about birth can all block the flow of labor.

Feelings of being a performer can impede the energy of birth and lead to lack of progress or failure of labor. This exercise is to help you explore your feelings concerning your performance during labor, breastfeeding and childcare.

Imagine each of the following situations, one at a time. First get into a state of deep relaxation. After imagining yourself, notice how you feel, what you hope you will do, what you wish others will think of you. After coming out of your state of relaxation, think about what it is that you truly value about childbirth, breastfeeding and childcare, and how it relates to the form these values ultimately (and practically) take, in everyday life.

Situation 1: You are in labor. Your labor and birthing is being filmed for use in your friend's natural childbirth classes. Your contractions are very difficult and seem to last forever, but your coach is telling you that you are doing a great job.

Situation 2: Everyone you know with children has easily breastfed them until they were two or three years old. You are at a party with some of these women, and your husband mentions that you plan to breastfeed for only six months so that you can more easily work outside of your home.

Situation 3: You are at the grocery store with your toddler. He or she has a temper tantrum over playing with everything within reach. You are tired and hungry and yell, "Shut up," slapping the small hand as it reaches one more time for the carton of eggs. Everyone is staring at you.

Key ways to avoid feeling like you have to perform are to stay in a relaxed and comfortable environment until labor is well underway. This means staying at home until your contractions are well within your doctor's recommendation for coming to the hospital. Or it means signing yourself out and going home if you arrive too early and labor stops. If you need someone to be with you at home so you feel comfortable about when to go to the hospital, find someone who can "labor sit." It's probably the best insurance you can find against a cesarean.

If you are birthing at home, it means paying attention to the environment and to whom you invite. You can alert everyone that your waters have broken or that you are having some contractions, but it is usually better not to invite people over until your labor is established. Make sure you feel comfortable or uninhibited with everyone present. If you are having photographs, you need to feel like you can throw them away afterward rather than being afraid of how you look!

Once at a home visit with a woman before her due date, there was a full spread of hors d'oeuvres and a party. Rahima suspected the woman was going to do the same thing during labor, so she didn't phone the other midwives or the woman's friends until she was at 8 centimeters. Then, despite the intensity of labor, everything stopped and the woman played hostess to quite a party. Who were the midwives to deprive her of this aspect of her birth! However, it was 4 a.m., and after an hour or so of no contractions, she remembered the birth and got discouraged that nothing was happening. Massage of her belly and nipple stimulation in the quiet of her bedroom soon brought contractions back strongly, and the baby was born within half an hour. Having to perform can take many forms!

Further Blocks to Energy in Labor

Lack of progress, failure of labor and cephalo-pelvic disproportion are catch-all terms indiscriminately put on charts during long labors to justify cesarean sections and/or pitocin followed by a cesarean. Real causes range from overcrowding or the doctor's need to hurry things along to a baby whose head is genuinely requiring extra time and effort to fit through the pelvis. The cause of a slowed labor can often be traced to a lack of understanding of the energy of birth and a failure to work with it. Unfortunately, most hospital personnel aren't even aware that such energy exists, let alone that it can be affected by their remarks, procedures and loving touch. Labor-and-delivery nurses have the possibility of being so much more helpful to women than they often are, due to lack of awareness, hospital policies and overcrowding. They never really know what it is like to go through labor and delivery with a woman—certainly not what birth is like in a setting that can allow for the full power of birthing energy without confinement by institutional policies.

Despite the changes of shifts, it is possible for nurses to give much more to laboring women through their touch, their warmth and their willingness to share emotionally with women when they are with them.

Lack of Progress

Lack of progress, uterine interia, failure of labor, or *dystocia* are all terms meaning that dilation of the cervix or descent of the head have been progressing too slowly or stopped altogether. It is uncommon for contractions to be very strong without progress, a condition that needs careful monitoring to prevent

thinning of the lower uterine segment or damage to the baby's head. Much more commonly, contractions remain far apart or are weak and ineffectual at dilating the cervix or bringing the baby down. Hence the prescribed treatments are pitocin to augment contractions, forceps and/or cesarean delivery.

The most frequent cause of lack of progress, one which is rarely recognized in hospitals, is a block in the energy of birth. The term *psychological dystocia* can be applied to many stalled labors, but this fails to include the interactive character of the mother and her environment. Midwives who work with birthing women know that it is frequently possible to go on to a successful delivery by helping the mother change her thoughts and feelings; other times it is possible, simply by changing her position or the environment, for the energy to pick up again.

Most birthing women receive the label *failure to progress* when their cervical dilation doesn't match the national average established by Friedman et al in 1957.[8] Barbara Katz Rothman, author of *In Labor: Women and Power in the Birth Place*,[9] points out that Friedman's curve, which plots dilation against hours in labor to define "normal labor," was formed by taking a statistical average of how long labors lasted. Then the *statistically* abnormal was equated with the *pathologically* abnormal. This is like saying if women on the average are 5'5" tall, then those who are in the minority (4'11" or 5'11") are sick and require medical intervention. No one would say this about the range of heights, but any *labor* which deviates from the norm is felt to require intervention to bring it back into line or to end it with cesarean section. Homebirth practitioners have found many common variations from Friedman's curve, including plateaus, a time of rest at full dilation, and the fact that early labor may stop and start (doctors call this false labor because normal labor *must* follow their curve without stopping and starting). Such variations have been pathological only insofar as they violated the timetable; outcomes were excellent.

Some tips for avoiding lack of progress or troubleshooting, should it happen to you:

● Rest during early labor. It can go on a long time before you get to 4 centimeters, and you'll need that energy for the end. Sleep or stay vertical (sitting or walking), depending on when it starts. Don't be "in labor" too soon.
● Keep up your energy by eating and drinking. You need that energy!
● Refuse routine fetal monitoring if your baby's

heartbeat is strong. Change positions often. Sitting, squatting and walking strengthen contractions and increase progress.

● Welcome the increasing intensity. Focus on the opening. Visualize. Say what you are doing. Surrender. Let it happen.

● Has anyone said anything that invalidated your progress? Speak about it. Is something only half overheard bothering you? Remarks of attendants can stop labor.

● Monitor the energy. Is anyone present who is afraid or negative? Is anyone making the mother tense? If so, ask them to leave. Find an important item for them to buy at an all-night drug store, or explain the situation to them. Would someone's arrival make the mother feel more secure? Is the energy being dissipated by too many people or by people being unfocused? In a homebirth, have a separate room where those present can eat, sleep or talk. Keep energy focused around the mother.

● In the hospital, you can go on as long as vital signs are good. Ask for a second opinion. Rally strength and get on with it.

● Change the environment. Can you become active, or could you rest? Would being alone with your partner be helpful? Would being entirely alone be worthwhile?

● Are you discouraged? Stay in present time. Know that labor and/or dilation can and will pick up again. Pretend that you just went into labor at this point. How would you feel? We once had a woman who had to imagine starting over three times during a long labor. She went on to a fine delivery.

● Resolve any inner conflicts. The most common revolve around:

  ● Medical/safety aspect. Are you where you need to be to give birth?

  ● Ambivalence about motherhood.

  ● Doubting that you can do it. But the baby will come out. It's going to be born one way or another, naturally, with forceps or with a cesarean. If you come to that realization and make a conscious choice to do it, you *will* be able to. Laugh, cry, swear, yell, change your energy.

  ● Lack of commitment. Do you really want anesthesia or a cesarean? You didn't before. What if you were alone? You'd have the baby just fine. Remember your resolve.

  ● Sometimes lack of harmony between a woman and her husband can impede labor. Is there anything you need to say to each other, or should he go out for a while?

Any change, in the people, the environment, the mother's position or her emotional state, will often enable labor to resume. Attendants who are sensitive to women and labor can go a long way to help avoid blocks in the energy. Focusing with the mother, monitoring the environment, letting her talk if necessary, helping her into other positions, encouraging her with words and with loving touch, all can be of tremendous help in preventing cesareans.

Almost every woman would keep labor at bay and not let it be strong if she could have her baby that way. But it isn't possible. You have to welcome its increasing intensity and let it come.

Cephalo-Pelvic Disproportion

"CPD" means the baby's head and the mother's pelvis are mismatched. If this really occurred as often as the label is applied to women's charts, the race would have ended long ago. In fact, it is used synonymously with "failure of labor" and "lack of progress" and has very little relationship to a woman's pelvic size or ability to birth. This is born out by the numerous cases of VBAC women giving birth to larger babies than the ones for which they had cesareans.

Any remark that a gynecologist or obstetrician makes about a "small pelvis" or "prominent spines" or "such a large baby" prior to two hours of pushing does nothing but undermine confidence and contribute to the high cesarean rate. It is impossible to predict and foolish to worry during pregnancy about whether or not a baby will come out vaginally. The reasons are that even with ultrasound, which can be inaccurate or misinterpreted under the best of circumstances, no one can predict how much the baby's head bones will overlap or mold during labor, how strong the contractions will be, and how much the mother's pelvic ligaments will relax and open during labor under the influence of the hormone relaxin and the pressure of the baby's head. Just a straight squat measurably increases the pelvic diameter, but how many doctors are willing to let a mother squat to deliver?

Undue concern about first babies, including requiring x-rays because the mother's pelvis is "untried," is another thing which serves only to undermine women's confidence in their ability to give birth. Keep your confidence, mother-to-be. Your body was made to have babies, and it will do so. The Farm in Tennessee gives us some idea how little the term CPD might be used if attendants worked with the energy instead. Farm midwives have delivered more than 1200 babies, most of them at home, and have had a cesarean rate of 1.5 percent compared to 18 to 20 percent nationally and 33 to 45 percent at some large teaching hospitals. They have had *one* case of cephalo-pelvic disproportion. You're no different from every other woman who has given birth!

Various Women's Dialogues About Blocks to Birthing Energy (B.E.)

Me: *How will you manifest yourself?*
B.E.: *In ways individual to everyone.*
Me: *But what about me?*
B.E.: *However you make me, I'll be.*
Me: *So I need to be open?*
B.E.: *If you wish. It will lead to a more pleasant experience.*
Me: *How do I open to you?*
B.E.: *By relaxing; accepting the flow; connecting with the baby; looking inward to your self, your soul.*
Me: *How do obstructions to the flow happen?*
B.E.: *When people won't accept me for what I am; when they don't acknowledge me as a real presence at a birth; when people or things with negative energies are present.*
Me: *How do I prevent it?*
B.E.: *By knowing yourself—your wants, desires, feelings; your headspace.*
Me: *How do I do that?*
B.E.: *Look inward, be in touch with yourself, listen to your heart.*

♦

B.E.: *Ready.*
Me: *Well, I'm trying.*
B.E.: *Don't be frightened. I am here to help you get your baby out to be with you.*
Me: *I know this . . .*
B.E.: *But still you're troubled.*
Me: *Yes.*
B.E.: *How can I help?*
Me: *You can't. You are doing your job. I should help you.*
B.E.: *OK. Relax. Think baby. Think opening.*
Me: *That's all?*
B.E.: *Yes. Working together is the key. I don't hurt you in anger. It is a part of my job of contraction and pushing your baby out to see you.*
Me: *I love you for that. Thank you, Birthing Energy. I am glad we work together.*

♦

B.E.: *Things are really intense.*
Me: *(an attendant): Yes, but we are all staying in touch with it.*
B.E.: *There is a new entity that is sapping and not contributing to me.*
Me: *I will deal with this now.*
B.E.: *I am peaking and focused again.*
Me: *Feels really good.*

B.E.: *Birthing energy is self-centered.*
Me: *Do you mean selfish?*
B.E.: *No, but it focuses on your body and your baby and everything else should be secondary.*
Me: *But I really want to share this experience.*
B.E.: *That's fine, but you can give them the best gift by taking their energy and letting them look to their own needs. This is no time to play Supermom or Superhostess. Allow the people you love to support and nurture you. Don't feel you're giving them a performance.*

What If You Birthed Alone?

We are not advocating childbirth without prenatal care and a skilled attendant! But we met a woman once who had given birth at home, entirely alone. She hadn't planned it that way, but she ended up having the baby without anyone else present. We met her four months after the birth, and she was still assimilating the fact that she had done something entirely impossible. That fact had completely transformed and empowered her. Although she didn't feel that other women should give birth alone, her question was a valid one: Why is it never mentioned that a woman *could* give birth alone? In childbirth education classes we talk about cesarean sections, but never about a woman's ability to birth with only her own power. Why is that any scarier to contemplate than a cesarean?

So this exercise is dedicated to her. We also want to include something you never hear about, because you never meet anyone who has birthed entirely without intervention. She said that the energy connection between her and her baby was incredible the whole time, as if the baby were directing her. She felt that anyone's presence would have really interrupted that.

Imagine birthing alone. What are your first reactions? What do the key words tell you?

_____

_____

_____

_____

_____

On whom are you most dependent? "I couldn't do it without . . ."

_____

_____

_____

Right off the top of your head, why wouldn't it work? (Examples: "The baby wouldn't come out." "I'd bleed to death." "What about the cord?") What is your reaction? Does it say anything to you?

_____

_____

_____

Preventing Cesareans and Avoiding Repeat Cesareans

Because we feel that it's difficult to improve on the work of Nancy Wainer Cohen, founder of C/SEC and co-author of _Silent Knife: Cesarean Prevention and Vaginal Birth after Cesarean_,[10] we include this checklist with her permission.

Prevent cesareans, and avoid repeat cesareans by:

- reading consumer oriented materials
- being nutritionally aware and eating well
- exercising
- learning about medical interventions and their consequences
- understanding that a woman's belief about herself and her labor determine the course of that labor
- learning what beliefs and attitudes you bring with you to your birth
- finding a midwife or labor coach who believe in birth without intervention
- selecting a doctor who understands and supports your wishes (and with whom you can communicate freely)
- clearing out your past birth experience
- developing positive attitudes and beliefs
- designing a hospital request list
- getting really in tune with your spouse
- developing a network of support (to encourage and applaud you)
- getting in touch with your strength and ability to open up and give birth
- constantly thinking how lucky your baby is going to be—born _naturally!_
- practicing relaxation exercises
- practicing visualization techniques (and using these to learn about yourself)
- realizing that women for centuries have been able to give birth
- loving your pregnant body
- practicing touching and massage
- understanding that childbirth is a beautiful way to learn about yourself
- remembering that you can depend on people who love you and care about you during labor
- avoiding medical interventions
- avoiding psychological interventions
- remaining clear about what your needs and rights are
- stomping on your "mind parasites"
- preparing yourself physically, emotionally, psychologically, and spiritually
- remembering that your mind and your body work _together_
- keeping in mind you can help to create the kind of birthing environment you wish
- resting everyday so you don't go into labor exhausted
- expending the least amount of energy possible to get you through each contraction
- taking each contraction one-at-a-time
- remembering that you can eat lightly during labor

- changing positions (and scenery!)—or tuning into your psychological state—when labor slows down
- remembering that labor doesn't necessarily progress at an even tempo
- knowing when fear, tension, inhibitions, embarrassment, anger, etc., are affecting your labor
- remembering that some babies take their *time* to be born
- keeping in mind the couples in your class and the couples in classes before yours who care about you and are supporting you
- thinking "baby baby baby" during contractions
- using a *loving* focal point
- maintaining eye contact and touch contact
- forgetting your hang-ups about "transition"
- *not* thinking of labor as a performance
- going with your labor (doing whatever you need to do)
- realizing there is a "learning to labor" period
- remembering how safe VBAC is (pretend you are in Europe!)
- keeping in mind the baby's head need not be engaged
- letting this labor be its own unique experience—not your previous experience or a friend's experience
- learning, trusting, believing; trusting and feeling that you can do it.

You Can Do It!

You really can give birth. And you know it. We know it. Rahima was in Mexico briefly during the writing of this book and was amazed, once again, to see how many more pregnant women there are there. From ages sixteen to forty-five, they fill the streets. Rahima had to ask herself, "What's the big deal? Birth is so much a part of life. Why write book, anyway?"

But she went back and continued working on it with Terra. Even though you don't need to be clear to give birth and you don't need this book, we felt that there is a real difference between American women and their sisters in Mexico. Even though the physiology may be the same, the psyche and the ambience are not. In that culture, birth is commonplace, a part of life, and so is death. People live with both with much more immediacy than we do. Rahima's experience midwifing in Mexico was that they don't have the information or the hangups that Americans do, so in that sense perhaps they do birth more "naturally." But along with an acceptance of birth there seemed to be an unconscious attitude of "getting through it," in whatever way one did, because it was woman's lot.

Perhaps we as American women are too well-educated and too caught up in psychology, just as we are too enamored of technology. But our cesarean rate speaks to the fact that we have to acknowledge where we are and do something about it. We can't go "back" to natural childbirth, to just squatting and letting it happen. But we can come to a new consciousness and a new confidence about birth, and we can reclaim it for ourselves from the male practitioners and male models that have come to dominate it in this century.

Birth in developed Western nations is in a fine muddle, as the British would say, or is completely bonkers, as we might say. There must be a reclaiming of giving and attending birth by women, for their own and their children's sakes, and for the future of society. This book is offered to help restore your confidence in your ability to give birth and to remind you of your power as women.

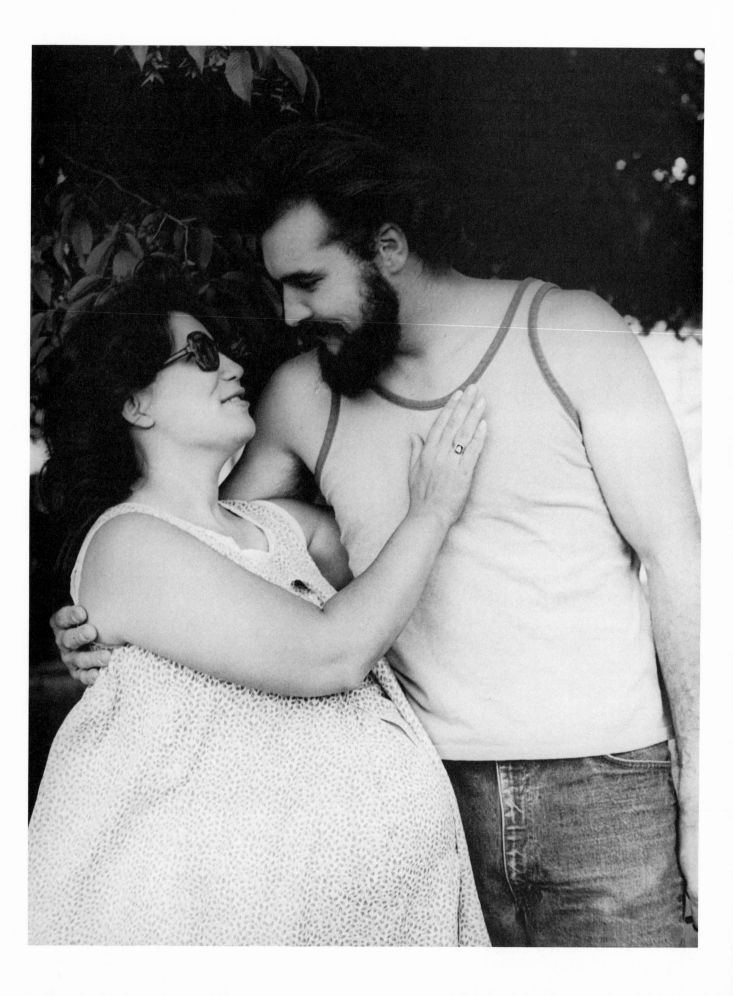

10
Looking Toward Parenting

Disagreement about rearing children can undermine a marriage. Actually, it is unconsciousness that is dangerous because disagreement can certainly be negotiated. But not knowing that you hold different viewpoints or are trying to accomplish different things can result in unnecessary suffering for all members of the family.

Many couples enter their marriage trying to be as aware as possible of male and female issues. They form agreements about attitudes, money, division of labor, and so forth. But the area of parenting often goes unexamined. Before the baby is born it is difficult for it to seem real or to know what the issues are. After the baby comes, parents keep adapting and coping as best they can, again often failing to recognize the issues. This chapter is designed to help you and your partner clarify your own values and ideals, and to communicate with each other about them.

The Ideal and the Real

Complete the following sentences with all the words that come to mind for you. Have your partner do it, too, and compare.

A mother is . . .

_____ _____ _____

_____ _____ _____

_____ _____ _____

_____ _____ _____

_____ _____ _____

_____ _____ _____

_____ _____ _____

_____ _____ _____

A father is:

_____ _____ _____

_____ _____ _____

_____ _____ _____

_____ _____ _____

_____ _____ _____

_____ _____ _____

_____ _____ _____

_____ _____ _____

A baby is:

_____ _____ _____

_____ _____ _____

_____ _____ _____

_____ _____ _____

_____ _____ _____

_____ _____ _____

_____ _____ _____

_____ _____ _____

_____ _____ _____

_____ _____ _____

_____ _____ _____

Now go back and think about your own mother and your own father, and add words to the lists. How did these words differ, if at all? What had you forgotten?

Now look at your lists and see what strikes you. Are there significant differences between father and mother? Do your list and your partner's differ significantly? Does a role as you have defined it include being all things to all people? Where in this description is there room for you? Where your list describes your own parents, do you want to be different as a father or mother? In what ways? Is it possible? How can our ideals be tempered with reality?

Roles as we see them often involve meeting the needs of others. It *is* possible to have your own needs met as a person while being a mother. The new environments of pregnancy and motherhood need not thwart our fulfillment, but may require some adjustment as to how we get our needs met. Fortunately, emotional needs can be met in many ways.

Meeting Your Needs

This exercise is to determine what needs are being met by the activities you do now, and then to think creatively of some new possibilities for achieving that same fulfillment through activities that fit in with the lifestyles of pregnancy and motherhood.

1. List some activities that are important to you.
2. Name the need(s) each fulfills.
3. Can you continue this activity during pregnancy/motherhood?
4. If not, name some alternative channels for fulfilling this need.

1. Activity	2. Need	3. Continue?	4. Alternatives

Issues of Parenting

This exercise is to familiarize you with some issues that come up during parenting. It will allow you to see which ones you need to learn about, which ones you already feel strongly about, and how your ideas coincide with those of your partner. React to each with an agree (+), disagree (−), or undecided (?). Have your partner do it too; then compare answers.

You Him
____ ____ Parenting is an instinctive skill.
____ ____ Babies should sleep in their own beds.
____ ____ Babies should have their own room.
____ ____ Breastfeeding is more convenient.
____ ____ Mothers should have the major childcare responsibility.
____ ____ Babies should sleep with their parents.
____ ____ It's OK to breastfeed in public.
____ ____ Boy babies should not wear pink clothes.
____ ____ You needn't talk to babies because they don't understand anyway.
____ ____ Boy babies shouldn't be circumcized.

You Him
____ ____ Vaccinations are necessary for children's good health.
____ ____ Everyone should be quiet when the baby is sleeping.
____ ____ Babies need to wear clothes in the summer.
____ ____ Commercial baby food is nutritious for babies.
____ ____ Breastfeeding should continue as long as the baby wants.
____ ____ Parents should not make love in the same room with the baby.
____ ____ You shouldn't pick up a baby every time it cries.
____ ____ Babies need baths every day.
____ ____ Pacifiers are not good for babies.
____ ____ Disposable diapers are not good for babies.
____ ____ When children can walk they are no longer babies.
____ ____ Babies can not be spoiled.
____ ____ Children should not be spanked.
____ ____ Babies should be baptized.
____ ____ Children should be weaned from bottles by one year of age.
____ ____ The first nine months of life the baby should be close to a parent at all times.

Feminism and Motherhood

Just as the feminist self-health movement has encouraged women to rediscover and lay claim to their own bodies, so too can a woman-centered point of view help women to reclaim the feminine power of birth. This power has been suppressed, diverted and denied by medical practices designed to "save us" from pain, from our own bodily functions, and from midwives, who have traditionally been the guardians of normal birth.

However, there are people who call themselves feminists who have themselves belittled motherhood and giving birth, perhaps out of hatred for men, the fear of becoming like their own mothers, or wanting to avoid the isolation and dependence often experienced by mothers in our culture. When Rahima was pregnant with her first child in 1973, she eagerly went into the newly opened feminist book store asking for books on childbirth. She was promptly laughed out of the building. Fortunately, the feminist movement in general has come to realize that birth, as well as parenting, is an issue worthy of concern and integral to the evolution of society and each individual in it.

The realities of parenting today are much different from even a generation ago for people in the United States. In 1980, only 28 percent of all families were made up of an employed father and a fulltime homemaker-mother. Not many of us have come to fulfill the *Father Knows Best* and Donna Reed models of family life offered to us on TV in our childhoods. In 1982, women made up 43 percent of the labor force in our country, with 40 percent of their children in home daycare with a sitter and another 40 percent in family daycare with four to six other children in a sitter's home. About 45 percent of the women employed outside of the home were single (divorced, widowed, never married) and self-supporting with dependent children. Of the over 8 million women raising children alone, only 59 percent had been awarded any child support and of those, 72 percent actually received any payment, with only 47 percent receiving the full amount.[1]

The economic and social conditions that led women to enter the labor force in large numbers coincided with the consciousness raising of feminism to encourage assertive seeking of equality in pay and advancement in work outside the home. Now, it seems, the time is right for us to demand recognition for work at home—childcare and housecleaning. In a reaction against the old values, many women have fallen into the trap of not valuing motherhood in the same way society undervalues motherhood and nurturing professions such as teaching, nursing and providing daycare.

Rahima feels that women need to come from a place of feeling lost as parents and even not wanting to be with their children, to having confidence in their own ability to mother and to value the time spent with young children. Such time tends not to be "goal-directed" and does not lead to tangible results on a day-to-day basis. But the presence of the mother makes a real difference in a child's life, especially in the first year. As a preschool teacher, Rahima has to report that the effects of children under three being with their mother only in evenings *is* tangible by the age of 5 or 6 and has a lasting influence on the individual and on society.

As more and more women enter the work force as single parents or necessary contributors to their family's finances, women find themselves trying to balance mothering and their children's needs with jobs or careers. Sometimes it is possible to work within the home, provide daycare, or figure out other ways of having your child with you while you earn money. Terra emphasizes that we need to teach our children the diversity of roles that may be possible for them as adults. Why train girls to be Donna Reed when probably less than 28 percent of them will get to do that? Why not train boys to be nurturing fathers who will take an active role in caring for their own children?

It is important to explore the idea, realities and emotions connected to fathers taking an active role in child care. Babies have already spent nine months with their mothers before they are born. The association of mother with nurturance is further reinforced by breastfeeding. Some couples choose to express breast milk or give a formula for one or more of the baby's feedings so that the father can feed the baby too. Although this practice does not coincide with the philosophy of La Leche League and many other groups associated with natural childbirth, each of us needs to adapt to our own values the life situation we are creating for our children. (There is a rumor from several different sources that it is possible for men to breastfeed. This would certainly revolutionize the parenting process!)

Even if the father is limited in his nurturing of the baby with food, he can play an active role in other respects. The idea of *fathering* the child, rather than babysitting when the mother needs to do something else, can bring its own rewards. After all, we don't consider a mother to be babysitting her children; she is being their mother and seeing to their needs and growth.

There may also be a point in sharing the children, where the mother may not be able to let go of being the authority on the child—her traditional territory—so that the father feels free to grow in that direction. Just as with housework, where a woman often ends up doing more than a fair share because she can no longer stand the mess, she might find it more of a hassle to ask that things be done for the baby than to do them herself. Coming to a balance where you both feel comfortable involves awareness of power plays, as well as fairness and the actual needs of the baby. Bonding awareness by the father can go a long way in promoting a strong nurturing relationship between father and baby.

Some suggestions for sharing:

1. Start communicating prenatally about parenting and expectations each of you has about the role of the other.
2. Be sure that the father has lots of bonding time with the baby after the birth and beyond.
3. Leave the father alone with the baby.
4. When you are both with the baby, make it clear who is in charge at that particular time.
5. Encourage the father to develop a repertoire of actions that can help soothe the baby without a breast.
6. Include washing diapers as a task to be split, along with diapering itself.
7. Infant massage by the papa can encourage nonverbal communication between father and baby.

THE BEGINNING OF PATRIARCHY

women were part of creation.
we painted our faces with our moonly blood,
offered freely from deep in our bodies to
Mother Earth.
we painted our breasts with it.
our power flowed freely, as our blood did,
without struggle.
we did not hold power to ourselves, it was like
the ripe fruit falling from trees.
and when the blood did not come
it grew into a child with milk to feed the child.

the men could not offer blood so easily.
they did not bleed without danger.
their blood did not grow into children.
they began to hunt and sacrifice animal blood
and eat animal flesh to try to take the power
of the animals to themselves.
they cut themselves to bleed in imitation of us
women.
they began to pretend giving birth.
they made things and treated them better than
the children.
we watched them, not wishing them such pain.
they began to do their magic in secret from us.
they said the blood they offered was real blood,
their god wanted no women's blood.
their god wanted us to hide our blood as unclean
and not worship near men.
we did not understand why blood that makes life
and is given freely is bad and blood made of
death is good.

Terra

Child Care, Household and Financial Responsibilities

Optimal use of this exercise would be for you and your partner to react separately to these statements and then discuss your reactions. Note if you agree (+), disagree (–), or are undecided (?). (As with all of the exercises that explore feelings, we do not necessarily advocate these statements. They are listed to stimulate opinion and discussion.)

You	Him	
___	___	**It's natural for a woman to take care of children.**
___	___	**If a woman doesn't bring in pay, she should do all of the housework and childcare.**
___	___	**Household responsibilities should always be divided equally among adult members.**
___	___	**Financial responsibilities should always be divided equally between adult family members.**

You   Him

_____ _____   Because a woman must deal with
                sexist hiring practices and pay
                scales, her work time should count
                equally with her partner's work
                time when figuring how much
                each should contribute to family
                expenses.

_____ _____   Household and childcare services
                should be paid for, to whomever
                does them, by the spouse who is
                working outside the home, so that
                the house wife or house husband
                has her/his own money to contri-
                bute to family expenses and for
                personal use. (This is not an
                allowance.)

_____ _____   If one partner takes care of the
                yard, construction, mechanical and
                repair work, it's fair for the other
                to do all of the cooking, cleaning,
                and childcare.

_____ _____   Structured sharing of jobs work
                out better than *laissez-faire*
                methods which might cast one
                partner in the role of having to
                complain about the contributions
                of the other partner.

What do YOU Want?

Think about these subjects and discuss them
with your partner.

During Pregnancy:

Will you work at an outside job during pregnancy? How long? If not—how does this affect
sharing household and financial responsibilities?

_____

_____

_____

After the birth:

● How long will you remain at home with the
baby? Will you work outside the home after
six weeks? Six months? Three years? Five
years? You must balance your recovery needs,

baby's care needs, financial needs, and your
need for involvement with your baby and the
outside world.

_____

_____

_____

● Will you try to find work to do at home
that pays income, such as childcare, sewing,
typing, cottage industries, consulting work,
writing, telephone solicitation?

_____

_____

_____

● Will your partner share childcare responsibilities? Is it dependent on how much he
works outside of the home? Is his share
always 50/50? Will you rotate responsibilities?
Does childcare include washing diapers, feeding, bathing, getting up at night, shopping for
clothes, getting babysitters?

_____

_____

_____

● Will your partner share household responsibilities? Does his share depend on job situations? Is it half? Are responsibilities structured?

_____

_____

_____

● How old might your child be when first left
with a babysitter? What qualities do you want
in a sitter?

_____

_____

• If you do not get a personal income, how do you share money?

_____

_____

_____

Single Motherhood

It is becoming increasingly common for women to be the only parent raising one or more children, either intentionally or through divorce or abandonment of support. If this happens before the baby is born, it is important to have certain issues concerning the child's father as clear as possible. (These were discussed in Chapter 2.) It is also important for single parents to arrange adequate support for the birth and postpartum. Here we would like to have you focus on some of the aspects of being a single parent, if that is your situation.

The financial responsibilities of having to be primary or sole support for a family while having a baby or a young child can be difficult to juggle. How will you be supported? Will you go back to work or seek a job outside the home? Will you receive welfare or Aid to Dependent Children? Will you be able to work at home or take your baby to the job with you? Will that be possible when he or she becomes older?

If you don't have definite answers to these questions, brainstorm about possibilities. Don't worry about whether they are realistic or not. Maybe you will become inspired. Whom can you get to help you look for work or apply for aid?

Where will you live? Can you continue living where you are, or will the arrival of the child mean that you need to move? If you will be living with your parents, what are the advantages and disadvantages? Is it possible to live communally or with friends? What would be the possible trade-offs? Brainstorm about possible situations, such as a duplex with another woman who loves to babysit or offering room and board to someone in exchange for childcare, and so forth.

What are your short term and long term goals? What are your values in parenting, and how do these form and interact with your goals?

Where can you turn for support? Is there a friend or counselor you can talk to if the going gets rough?

Is there a friend or relative who is a parent whom you can ask for advice if your child is sick or you have questions about a new baby? Are you in touch with support groups such as La Leche League for breastfeeding or a single mother's group or parent support group?

What about your own social life? Do you have or foresee adequate opportunities for adult companionship? Can you meet people through a single parent's group or a religious or interest group?

What about childcare? Do you plan on taking your baby with you most places when it is very young? Are there any places that are inappropriate for a baby, which you would be better to give up? How old will your baby be before you will want occasional babysitting or regular childcare? Whom can you contact? The Department of Social Services usually makes referrals to licensed daycare homes, or there may be local daycare home associations. The demand for quality fulltime childcare for children under the age of two-and-a-half exceeds the supply.

What have we left out that is concerning you?

_____

_____

_____

_____

_____

"Elderly Primipara"

When a woman approaches thirty, she starts hearing phrases like "the biological clock is running out" or "elderly primipara" (ancient first-time mother). Such attitudes, especially from doctors, undermine a woman's confidence; the higher incidence of complications and cesareans may come from such expectations and from psychological ambivalence rather than any lack of stretch in the uterine tissues! Women have reproductive capacity well into their forties. If you are approaching thirty, we highly recommend one of the many workbooks dealing with pregnancy over thirty. You need to have all of the support, facts and confidence on your side to have a natural birth experience. We especially recommend *The Pregnancy After 30 Workbook* by Gail Sforza Brewer.[2]

If you are over thirty and this is your first baby (or there is a large gap between earlier children and this one):

1. Were there conscious reasons why you waited this long to have a child (or another child)? If so, then what were they? If not, then could you find any physical reason for the delay?

_____

_____

_____

2. What were the reactions you got from friends and family when you let them know you were pregnant? Do you think it would have been different if you had done it at an earlier age? How did these reactions sit with you?

_____

_____

_____

3. What are your fears, if any, about having a baby later in life?

_____

_____

_____

4. What are the advantages of having a baby later in life?

_____

_____

_____

5. Do you find your confidence and "at-home-ness" with your body has increased or decreased since you were 20 years old? Do you take more or less care of your body now than when you were younger?

_____

_____

_____

Your Parents

During pregnancy, men and women become more in touch with their own parents. Finally we experience what they went through! This can bring up strong feelings, buried since childhood, about their methods of dealing with us and about life in general. Remembering ourselves as children helps us to relate to our own children, and being a parent helps us relate to the difficulties and challenges our own parents had to face. We may gain new respect for the individuals who cared for us during our childhood, recognizing that they did their best at a difficult job. We might decide to do things differently than they did, but now we understand that the responsibility was heavy for them too. This may allow much resentment and anger towards our parents to fall away.

This exercise is to help you think about how your parents parented you, and how you felt, and still feel, about it. If this will be your first child, it might be interesting for you to repeat this exercise after two or three years of parenting and compare it with your responses during pregnancy.

Explore each listed topic with regard to your parents' efforts: put a "P" over the word that best describes their parenting. Compare your responses with those of your partner for an important and interesting conversation.

1. Style of discipline: authoritative—laissez faire—permissive—firm and consistent—other:

2. Showing affection: a lot—a little—just right—other:

3. Attitude towards money and property: most important—tools—useless—root of all evil—other:

4. Attitude towards one's body: evil and dirty—God's temple—to be enjoyed and used—indifferent—other:

5. Attitude towards sex: open and honest—secret—evil—sexually abusive—to be enjoyed—other:

6. Attitude towards strangers: friendly—ignore them—fear them—take advantage of them—other:

7. Attitude towards family members: close and loyal—tolerant—distant and hateful—distant and respectful—other:

8. Eating habits: forced to clean the plate—totally unstructured—junk food diet—nutrition conscious—other:

9. Did the family do things together: always—sometimes—seldom—other:

10 Support for individual activities (like sports, drama club, etc.): supported—ignored—discouraged—other:

11. Spiritual guidance: strict—delegated to the church or synagogue—encouraged personal exploration—none—other:

12. Educational/employment direction: pushed—encouraged—didn't care—discouraged—other:

13. Acceptance of your maturity: pushed it too early—encouraged—have not yet accepted it—other:

14. Attitude towards children in general: enjoyment—tolerance—ignore—other:

15. Attitude towards childbirth: miraculous—tolerable—disgusting—painful—other:

16. Attitude towards breastfeeding: encourage—tolerate—ignore—think it's impossible—think it's disgusting—other:

17. Communications within the family: clear—sarcastic—discouraged—unpleasant—indirect—open and honest—other:

18. Is there, or has there been, child abuse (physical or psychological) in your family of origin? (If so, please seek counseling, for what you experienced as a child may otherwise come up as you care for your own child.)

Are You the Same or Different?

Our parental behavior is determined by our own parents to an amazing degree. Either we unconsciously assume some of the same voice and habit patterns, or we decide to "do just the opposite." In either case, we are usually *reacting* rather than acting. And it is frustrating as a middle aged adult to see and hear ourselves manifesting precisely those traits of our parents that we most disliked.

This does not mean it isn't valuable to think about your ideals and values as parents. On the contrary it is extremely important. Most new parents today find that the rhythms, definitions and structures of traditional society are little help in defining parenting for them. People feel they need to learn how to parent. Learning involves experience, but also knowledge and forethought.

Return to the preceding exercise and put a "Y" over the words that best reflect your values in parenting.

You need to discuss with your partner such things as demand feeding, sleeping arrangements for the child (alone or in the family bed), discipline for the older child, authority, responsibility, immunization, schooling, and much more. But don't discuss your parenting with, or in front of, the children. Not only do your children need the sense that you both know and agree on what you are doing, but also they are better off unburdened by the issues of adult life. David Elkind, in *The Hurried Child,* points out the stress and other negative effects on children of involving them in discussions which are adult in nature.[3]

So do your discussing now, while your baby is still on the way or while your other children are asleep. Return to the last exercise and discuss how you would want to be with your own children, the same or different.

Friendships, Pregnancy and Mothering

When Terra found out she was pregnant she didn't have any friends who had given birth within the last ten years—all of her friends were either childless or had older children. Gradually, through childbirth classes and midwifery study groups, she came to know other women with small children who could relate to her magnificent obsession. You too might find your friendships shifting a bit with the coming of a baby.

That obsession with pregnancy and babyhood may be boring or alien to the lifestyle of some single friends. They might find it difficult to be around you if you alter your habits to suit your condition, such as quitting smoking or drinking alcohol. The blow-by-blow account of how often the baby has kicked you today just might not seem relevant to an outsider. And after the baby comes there is the rather constant interruption of conversation that occurs, not to speak of the sometimes disastrous effects of babies and toddlers on friends' white carpet and expensive bric-a-brac.

At the same time, some people without children are happy to participate in childrearing and will go out of their way to be a part of your child's life. These will be the friends who offer to babysit, and really do it. They will put fragile objects out of reach before the toddler arrives and they might even keep a few toys about for visiting children to play with.

Building a support network that includes people who have children around the same ages as yours will help you in your parenting efforts. You might even become friends with someone you normally wouldn't have chosen, just because your children get along so well.

1. How did your friends react to the news of your pregnancy? Were you surprised at their reaction? Did you express your feelings to them about their reaction?

_____

_____

_____

_____

_____

2. Has pregnancy affected any of your friendships? Has it been a positive or detrimental change?

_____

_____

_____

_____

_____

Responsibility

Pregnancy and parenthood are times to develop the ability to respond to situations as needed: "response ability." Responsibility is not achieved through rigid rules but through the flexibility and knowledge to deal with changes as they occur. The truth of this be-here-now attitude of parenthood first becomes evident as labor begins—usually at an unpredicted moment. After the birth, as the baby begins to exhibit its own unique personality, all schedules for sleep, food, and development fall by the wayside because they are only useful _averages_. "Response ability" requires knowledge of a range of possibilities, and sensitivity to the real situation that presents itself.

How do you react to responsibility?

_____

_____

_____

How do you respond? When something needs to be done, but you are busy, do you . . .
● **let it go until later?**
● **hope that someone else will do it?**
● **take the time to do it?**
● **other:**

Do you usually . . .
● **do what needs to be done?**
● **do it, while complaining?**
● **ask someone else to do it?**
● **tell someone else to do it?**
● **say, "It doesn't matter anyway"?**
● **say, "It's not my thing"?**
● **other:**

TIME FOR A CHANGE

We parents know when it's time for a change—
the preceding rumblings, grunts and grimaces,
the sweet odor, give it away.

sometimes we look at each other
waiting to see who will be the one to do the job.
none of us especially like to do it, when it's a big
    mess.
but when we don't—
that smell of aging poop
the oozing juices
rashes breaking out
and crying baby
tell us that it's better not to wait too long to
    make those changes.

This world sorely needs a new diaper.

                                                      Terra

Will You Breastfeed?

You need to decide during your pregnancy whether you will breastfeed. Perhaps you know that mother's milk is best suited for the baby, and that breastfeeding is easier, prevents allergies, and has a score of other advantages. Even if all your friends have breastfed their babies and there has never been a doubt in your mind, read *Special Delivery* or a manual on breastfeeding and contact La Leche League for monthly meetings and the resource of telephone counselling. Common discomforts in the first few days—such as engorgement, sore nipples, or a baby who doesn't want to suck—can lead to serious problems if supplementary bottles are given. You need to be informed yourself, as well as to find a doctor who *actively* encourages breastfeeding.

It is good to know that you can nurse your baby even under special circumstances—everything from prematurity to a breast infection, or even an adopted baby! Get your resources (people and books) together now. They will mean a lot more to you when you need a quick answer while your baby is screaming.

In planning to breastfeed, it is important to see that your nipples stick out during pregnancy when they are stimulated or cold. Some women have inverted nipples, which can be corrected by wearing

special "Swedish milk cups" inside your support bra during pregnancy. You don't want to wait until your baby's birth day to find out that he or she can't latch on to your nipple!

Talk to your partner about breastfeeding. Were you or he breastfed? What do you feel about women breastfeeding in public places?

_____

_____

_____

_____

_____

What do you know of your mothers' attitudes towards breastfeeding? What have your sisters' or friends' experiences been?

_____

_____

_____

_____

_____

If you are questioning your ability to breastfeed, what is it that concerns you? How do you know that, or where did you get the idea? Are there other facts you can get? Is there another opinion of yourself you could have?

_____

_____

_____

_____

_____

_____

A small number of women say, "I'm too nervous to breastfeed." While it is true that the "let-down reflex" can be affected by nervousness, you can also learn what is bothering you and let it go. Any woman can nurse her baby, given the proper knowledge and support. What doubts or fears do you have?

_____

_____

_____

_____

If you had trouble nursing a previous baby, can you find out enough to know why it didn't work (a hovering grandmother; being separated from a premature baby and not being helped to express milk; tension; aversion to physical contact; other). If you want to breastfeed this time, how can you let go of those feelings and arrange better support for after the birth?

_____

_____

_____

If you don't want to breastfeed because of job commitments, could you breastfeed for the first few days? The colostrum, before your milk comes in, provides the baby with many weeks of passive immunity to diseases; it also helps to stimulate digestion. Could you breastfeed for a few weeks or months? Could you contact La Leche League and ask how working mothers manage to express and freeze their milk so their babies can have it during the day and they can nurse when they are home? It's like bonding, in which any increased time together is beneficial. Any amount of breastfeeding is better than none!

_____

_____

_____

If you have decided not to breastfeed, what are your reasons? How do you feel about that decision? Do you feel undermined by your mate, friends, or books like these? Remember that you are just as good a mother, and much of the emotional and physical closeness which occurs during breastfeeding can still go on if you bottle feed attentively. A baby takes in more than milk; it also feeds on the mother's attention, love and flow of energy. If you are bottle feeding, don't prop up a bottle and go away, feeling that you have handled your baby's needs.

_____

_____

_____

_____

_____

_____

◆   ◆   ◆

MOTHER'S MILK

my breasts ache and leak when my baby
  dreams of eating.
how can I give him rubber and glass?
how can I imagine him sucking a cow's udder?
or nuzzling a can of Similac?

Terra

◆   ◆   ◆

Will You Circumcize Your Baby?

If your baby is a boy, you will have to decide whether to have him circumcized. Most hospitals want you to sign the consent forms when you pre-register, so it pays to discuss this in advance with your mate.

Respond to the following statements with agree (+), disagree (−), or unsure (?). Have your partner do the same and then compare and discuss.

You Him

___ ___ **1. Circumcision represents an important religious covenant for our family.**

___ ___ **2. Babies don't feel any pain during circumcision.**

___ ___ **3. It's important to the grandparents that the baby be circumcized.**

___ ___ **4. Both parents should be present during the operation.**

___ ___ **5. Other children might make fun of him if he isn't circumcized.**

___ ___ **6. Other children might make fun of him if he is.**

___ ___ **7. Boys should be the same as their father and brothers.**

___ ___ **8. If he isn't circumcized he's likely to get adhesions and need to be circumcized as an adult; better now than then!**

___ ___ **9. There are no medical reasons for circumcision.**

___ ___ **10. There are no risks involved in the operation.**

___ ___ **11. If he isn't circumcized, the foreskin should not be pulled back for the first year.**

___ ___ **12. Circumcized men are better lovers.**

___ ___ **13. Uncircumcized men have a lower incidence of cancer.**

You need the facts as well as looking at your own emotional and irrational beliefs. The American College of Pediatricians has just issued a statement that the foreskin should *not* be pulled back on uncircumsized babies. We recommend the books *Circumcision: An American Health Fallacy* by Edward Wallerstein[4] and *Circumcision: The Painful Dilemma* by Rosemary Romberg.[5]

As in all other areas, we suggest that you inform yourself and make conscious and responsible decisions. If you are going to have your baby boy circumcized, know why you are doing it and be present during the operation or ceremony. What's the point of a conscious and intentional birth followed by an unthought-through surgery?

Lessening Family Rivalry

The arrival of a new baby means spending a lot of time and energy with this new being. Other members of your family (even pets) may feel a little displaced and it can seem that there's not enough of Mom to go around! Your husband may also be feeling at a loss due to your preoccupation with the baby. Even though he may welcome the new baby, there may be feelings of jealousy that you are more involved with the new baby than he is, or that the baby is getting all your attention. This is more common if you are always exhausted, emotional or out of sorts.

It is not surprising that a feeling of being displaced can occur after the birth, especially with a first baby, when the spontaneous life of couplehood must give way to include a new family member—24 hours a day! This adjustment can be especially trying for a relationship where the woman has been mothering the man, or lavishing all of her attention on him rather than pursuing her own outside interests. He may react with irritability, withdrawal or anger. With close communication you may be able to deal with situations like this, before the child is born. Be attentive to his moods, and ask what is bothering him.

In the case of a second or later child, the children already there must accept having another baby who will receive a lot of mom's and dad's attention.

Some suggestions for lessening sibling rivalry:

● Children love babies. Relate to this quality in them.

● Include everyone in planning, preparation, birth and bonding, childcare, etc. If you are not birthing at home, will your children be able to visit you often, or can you sign out early to shorten the time of separation?

● Get everyone to start relating to the baby before the birth.

● Plan a birthday party when the baby is born. Include a special toy or doll that your other child can mother.

● Be clear in yourself as to how much energy you put into your relationship with each family member.

● Before the birth, gradually "wean" a dependent person, being sure to spend some real time together regularly.

● Don't treat the baby as a precious object. Let other children hold and touch the baby freely (with supervision). Relax. Say "no" only when needed—then be really clear about it.

● Let your children help with things you need postpartum. Also arrange for special times for them so you can rest (e.g. a friend could take your toddler to the park).

● If necessary, seek family counselling in a difficult situation.

Postpartum Self-Care

The period of time after your baby has been born is one of love, activity and excitement. Yet it is a time when you need to rest and be with your family. And you need to eat really well, so that you can recover your energy. Not taking care of yourself postpartum can take its toll later.

Try to arrange to *stay in bed for at least one week* (preferably two), and stick by it. We don't want to prescribe new "rules," but the tendency to overdo it is so common. Be in touch with your body, and remember that postpartum hemorrhage is most common between days 10 and 17. Keeping your legs together will help any small abrasions and any stitched episiotomies or tears to heal back into their normal positions more quickly. Pelvic floor exercises (see Chapter 7) will get the circulation going and thus promote healthy tissues, as well as toning all of the muscles that keep your pelvic organs in place and preventing accidental urine loss when coughing. Gentle exercise programs are heartily recommended; see the Appendix for several books with suggestions.

To stay in bed two weeks might seem like a lot, but too much exertion too soon can lead to poor healing of the placental site, with delayed postpartum hemorrhage, incomplete healing of tiny vaginal tears, or even uterine prolapse. Be especially careful not to lift anything heavier than your newborn for at least six weeks to avoid uterine prolapse (including toddlers—have them climb up to you on a chair or have someone else lift them up to you). If you have bleeding after your discharge has become brown, you're doing too much!

Remember, you'll be adjusting to a new baby's feeding and waking schedule. Sleep when the baby sleeps—let the house be a mess if there's no one else around to clean it. The baby and your own rest are more important.

When friends or family members ask what they can do to help, don't be shy—have ready a list of things you need and enlist their aid. Some especially helpful shower gifts are: diaper service for a month or more; services of a mother's helper/housekeeper; lunches and/or dinners catered by friends or professionals for the first few weeks; and special little gifts or excursions and visits for older siblings of the new baby.

The psychological adjustments of new motherhood (even for experienced mothers) can be greater than you anticipate. The postpartum period is one that is often ignored during pregnancy, perhaps with the wish that it will disappear if we don't talk about it. The beauty of new love with a new baby is balanced by the practicalities of recuperating from labor, interrupted sleep, new roles to play, new division of time and energy, breasts not yet accustomed to breastfeeding, new skills to learn with a first baby or caring for several children without neglecting any of them, and maintaining a relationship with one's partner. Add a flurry of visiting grandparents and guests, and you have an idea of the possible pandemonium of postpartum. It's best to have at least thought and talked about how having the baby will effect the lives of each family member, individually and as a group. The exercises in this book bring up many of the relevant issues. Another excellent resource for guidance in this area is *Mothercare* by Lyn DelliQuadri and Kathi Breckenridge.[6]

Some practical tips we've learned by experience, and from our teachers and students, include:

● Be sure to have your household well-stocked and as clean as possible the last few weeks before your due date so that, right after the birth, shopping and cleaning won't be as necessary.

● Try a diaper service for the first month or two. It will save time and energy when you need to be taking it easy, and it is usually cheaper than disposable diapers.

● For first time parents who have not had experience around babies, a parenting class or help from a friendly couple who have a baby can be invaluable. Guidance in such skills as diapering, bathing the baby, putting on a baby carrier, choosing the best brands and so forth can make the postpartum period much easier to cope with. Parenting is a skill, so do not expect to do everything perfectly at first.

● Remember to make arrangements to stay home and in bed as much as possible for one or two weeks, without the need to do housework, cooking, shopping or laundry. Friends and family can often take care of these things, and in some communities there are services at a reasonable price for postpartum mothers.

● Try to pay your doctor or midwife before the birth if possible. There are more pleasant things to think about postpartum than paying bills.

● If you are going to have your older children be present, be sure to prepare them before the birth as much as possible. A helpful book is *Children at Birth* by the Hathaways.[7] Be sure to include children in the bonding process, and allow them to help as much as they are able. Also allow them to mourn the change, without pushing them away from you and the baby. Help them express their feelings in constructive ways.

● Educate yourself about what is normal for newborns and what to watch for. Start collecting information about such topics as circumcision, rooming-in for hospital birth, immunizations. Learn CPR and other first aid techniques, and you will be better able to deal with emergencies.

● Rest. It will make dealing with anything that comes up easier.

● Relax. It will help you keep centered through all of the changes.

● Enjoy. Keep your sense of humor and just let yourself fall in love with your new baby.

● Try to set up a support system before the birth.

Include other friends who are parents, people from your childbirth class, La Leche friends, family members.

● Pamper yourself as much as possible.

● Pamper your partner as much as possible.

● Get some fresh air and some time alone daily. Try to walk around the block as a first venture.

● Set priorities. Take care of yourself, the baby, and the family, then turn to laundry, cleaning, and other tasks.

● Focus on your particular religious or spiritual path and make use of the strength and nurturance that come to you from it.

● Arrange for someone to come and give you massage or other body work during the first few days postpartum. You'll feel so much better so much sooner!

● Don't deny your own feelings. Arrange to have someone come who will listen to your account of labor and delivery and help you release any unexpressed emotion. Keep your journal, your perspective and your sense of humor.

These are the major points of preparation. Can it be true that "In some 250 cultures of the world, the postpartum parent receives more adequate physical and emotional support than in the West?"[8] Be kind to yourself and arrange adequate support!

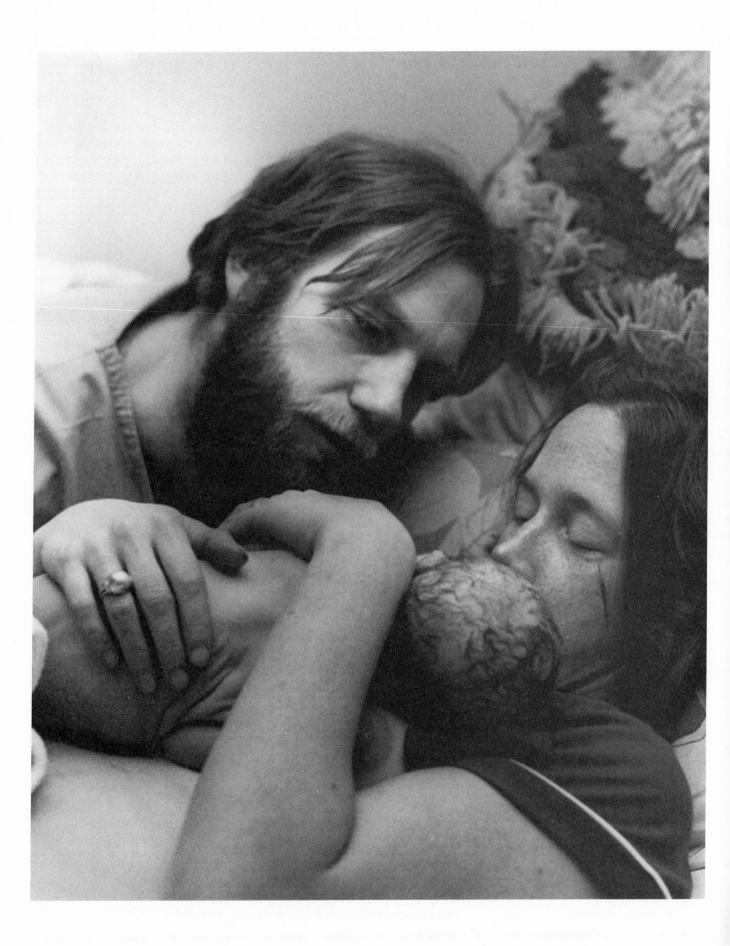

11
For New Parents
Integrating the Birth

In the days following a birth, everything seems to be enveloped in a special energy. It is a very special time to be together as parents and as a new family. It is always amazing to leave a home where a birth has occurred and find the rest of the world still much the same. Wordsworth describes this special energy surrounding a baby in his *Intimations of Immortality*:

Our birth is but a sleep and a forgetting:
The Soul that rises with us, our life's Star,
Hath had elsewhere its setting,
And cometh from afar:
Not in entire forgetfulness,
And not in utter nakedness,
But trailing clouds of Glory do we come
From God, who is our home:
Heaven lies about us in our infancy![1]

While that's something difficult to see, being open to the miracle of birth makes it possible for you to experience its higher quality. Because birth involves a very "high" or "intense" energy, it is good in the first few days to remember the details of labor and delivery and thus connect them with your normal consciousness. The amnesia of birth is well-known, and usually refers to the fact that women don't remember the discomfort of birth. But your body remembers everything, even if your mind doesn't, and the more you can bring your consciousness to the event, the less will remain to be cleared in the future.

Women love to talk about their births, but pay some attention to your body before you muster your postpartum consciousness to relive the labor and delivery. You have just been through an amazing physical experience, and having your body touched will help it to reintegrate and seem like "yours" again. If you have any friends who do massage, polarity, Touch for Health, energy balancing, or other body work, arrange in advance for them to come over in the first few days following the birth. Even if you have to pay for body work, the investment will be small in comparison to how much better you feel and how much more quickly you recover your strength.

Then arrange a time in which you can go through your birth experience with a friend who will sit and listen without interrupting you (follow the directions on page 62). Start wherever you feel labor began and relive the labor and delivery. Include any postpartum experiences that seem relevant. Allow whatever emotions are present to well up as you see and hear all that was said.

As a midwife, Rahima did this with her clients, who found it extremely helpful. As a midwife she could sometimes provide facts that helped the mother better understand something that happened, or she could make recommendations about ways of working with unresolved feelings.

See if there are more facts you can find out about anything in your birth that was out of the ordinary. You may be worried because the cord was around the baby's neck; checking with your attendant will help to clarify that this is common at births and probably posed no problem for your baby. Or you may find out what happened prior to your fainting, such as getting up too quickly. Feel free to ask your doctor or midwife any questions, and request a copy of your birth records. That way, if you move before your next birth you will have the records for your new attendant. This is especially valuable in the case of homebirths.

If you found areas of unresolved emotion in recounting your birth, think of ways of releasing it. Can you express your feelings to the person involved? Can you write to him or her? You might want to start one to your husband: "Some things I haven't told you about the birth . . ." Or you might want to tell a nurse that her remarks, though probably well-meaning, hurt your feelings. Use the techniques discussed in this book to release trapped energy before it has a chance to set into concrete. This is especially necessary if you had unexpected complications, but is also valuable for the "little things."

We found many unsuspected things surfaced when doing this exercise postpartum with women. Not all births required further inner work! Often we could just sit back and listen to a woman realizing her own growth and power through her experience of giving birth—for re-experiencing the birth can be very empowering.

Coming to peace with a birth experience is sometimes easy and sometimes not. This depends not only on what happened, but also on the woman herself. It is possible to feel good about a very difficult birth, while other times something seemingly minor can have a great deal of emotional charge behind it due to past loss or hurt. Grieving, forgiving, accepting are all appropriate for anything as momentous as giving birth; whatever it takes to get you there, do it. Don't feel that because you have a healthy baby and you had a "normal" birth you shouldn't be feeling the way you do. Attitudes like that got you where you are today!

Integrating a birth experience can take a few days or several months. Rahima was once approached by a woman whose birth she had attended many months earlier. The woman hadn't gone into labor for several days after her waters broke and she progressed very slowly for a second baby. When it was finally realized what she needed to feel supported, she opened up and went from 6 centimeters to crowning in two contractions. She was stunned to be holding her baby so suddenly. Rahima listened to her musings and finally said, "You know, Linda, there's always going to be an element of surprise in your birth, no matter how many times you go over it or try to get rid of it." At that point she released and accepted her birth experience as it was, for she had indeed been trying to make sense of that element of surprise.

Postpartum Images

What images are you living out postpartum? Many women unconsciously try to play Pioneer Woman, strong as a horse, stubborn as a mule. Because a woman is not sick after giving birth, they think they ought to be able to do everything from household management to shopping a few days postpartum. Be advised that the placental site is quite large and open until the uterus shrinks down to a more normal size. The most common times for postpartum hemorrhage are days 10 to 17, and the cause is usually over-exertion. If this is your movie, how can you be more responsive to slowing down, taking it easy, and accepting others' help?

Another scenario involves Poor Me, with tremendous feelings of loneliness. You have just returned from the hospital or everyone has gone home after a wonderful homebirth, your husband is back at work, everything is a mess, and you feel exhausted. While postpartum depression is nowhere near as common or strong when the woman consciously gives birth rather than having it done to her, the combination of hormones, tiredness, interrupted sleep and all the other necessary adjustments can seem overwhelming at times.

Other women can't stand attention or feeling pampered. They dutifully stay in bed but grit their teeth through all of the attention. They feel bored and hate ''being treated like an invalid.''

There are other scenarios as well. Think about how you are feeling after the birth. Exaggerate it into a soap opera script. What alternatives exist? How can you arrange to recuperate and enjoy it?

_____

_____

_____

_____

_____

Mothering the Mother

What if we had more positive images for our postpartum experience? In some cultures the mother is honored and waited on for forty days. She is massaged, touched and held by the older women, i.e. she is mothered while she is mothering her baby. In Mexico the forty days with each child are the only ''vacation'' that a mother ever gets—ignore the fact that the Church considers her unclean until a special mass is said. In certain subcultures in India, a trained woman comes and joins the family for the

forty days, taking care of the woman and other members of the family, so she is really free to be with the baby. Some women in America are beginning to appreciate the fact that there might be a specialness to the time immediately following the birth and are waiting a month or so before taking the baby out or going to meetings or social engagements themselves. They are trying to put their energy into the family without outside distractions during that time.

We've talked about the importance of lining up sufficient help for the postpartum period. If you are a brand new parent, how are you doing with this? Do you keep a list by the phone of things that are needed so you can suggest what callers can do to help? Do you feel harried, as if there are too many visitors? Can you bring some order into your days at home, resting when the baby sleeps and postponing things that are making you feel pressured?

Sometimes you have to mother yourself— certainly in the sense of looking after your own health and nutrition. Nurture yourself with adequate calories, rest, and the same amount of vitamins you were taking during your pregnancy. Nothing can be worse for you than crash dieting postpartum! Some women actually get on the scales after their birth, which is a real tyranny of the scales! Remember that you will be about the same size postpartum as you were at five months of pregnancy. That pair of favorite pants still won't fit. You need time to recover and sufficient energy for lactation. Breastfeeding burns up about 1000 extra calories a day, so if you eat nutritious food and watch the sweets, your weight will gradually come down.

Gradually resuming exercise can also make you feel better. Begin pelvic floor exercises the first day postpartum, and mild abdominal strengthening exercises can also be begun early. A good postpartum series of exercises is illustrated in _Special Delivery,_ and there are several programs on records or tapes available for pregnancy and postpartum. One of the advantages of a prenatal exercise class is that you not only form friends and a support group, but you're often welcome to return with the baby and exercise after the birth.

Your body is very different following a birth than it was before you were pregnant. Some women feel as if they are all breasts; others are excited to have a prominent bustline for the first time in their lives. Your hips and stomach will probably be rounder. You may have stretch marks. You may find that jogging makes you feel like your insides are falling out, or that your vagina sucks in air when you do a shoulder stand. Your vaginal area and cervix look different too. Clothes can be a problem, since you're tired of maternity clothes but nothing else fits. Remember that your body is still in transition, and will be as long as you are breastfeeding. Have patience, be abiding, and enjoy this time. It is limited in duration, and probably won't occur very many times in your life.

If you are reading this after the birth of your baby, draw a picture here of how you feel about your body:

The Emotional Rollercoaster

A woman who has just had a baby is tremendously open, both physically and emotionally. Having just been in touch with the full power of creation, she is aware of the vulnerability and frailty of life. A new mother taking her baby out on a walk for the first time cannot help feeling protective of this new being, wanting to shield him or her from the hazards of crossing streets or the noise and pollution of busy city life. A new mother may feel tremendously sad at the wilting of a flower or burst into tears of joy at the beaming face of a three-year-old. Such emotions are normal and are not a sign of postpartum depression, the baby blues or general craziness.

A woman's increased feeling of vulnerability can be helped when people around her are as considerate as possible. For example, if her husband is going to be half an hour late, a simple phone call can prevent unnecessary anxiety about accidents on the highway and being left alone with a newborn.

You will probably find your emotions are very fluid in the first days after birth. Just as your body has had to assimilate all of the sensations of giving birth, now you must also integrate all of the emotions that come so strongly. You may be elated, exhausted, excited, afraid and sad in rapid succession, or even all at the same time. Take the time to write in your journal a record of your thoughts and feelings during the first few weeks after your baby is born.

A feeling of sadness or grieving can enter in, even if you have had the most ideal birth. While having a new, healthy baby is very exciting, you have also lost some things as well. For one thing, you are no longer pregnant, and you may miss all of the attention, help and support that came to you then. You have also lost some of your personal freedom if this is your first baby; having to be aware of another person's well-being twenty-four hours a day is a real stretch for most people. You have also lost your old relationship as a couple, if this is your first baby. While you are now a family, which is what you wanted, the realities of decreased mobility, having to pack diaper bags or get babysitters, or a baby who invariably wakes up in the middle of lovemaking can remind you that things have indeed changed.

There can also be grieving if your baby is different from what you had imagined. If it is not the sex you had hoped, if he or she is very different from your other children—and certainly if there are any problems such as prematurity or congenital abnormalities—there is the need to integrate the fantasy baby with whom you have shared your body with the real baby you now have. Sometimes this integration is easy; other times it involves a real loss or letting go in order to come to terms with what is. We will deal with facing complications at the end of this chapter, but even such "minor" things as having a boy instead of a girl or vice versa can be cause for dismay. Write or tell someone about it; you're not a "bad mother" for feeling those things. Allow yourself to grieve, feel it fully, and allow the feelings to change.

There can also be a feeling of loss if your birth wasn't just the way you wanted it. This may be due to physical complications, the intervention of attendants, or impossible standards you set for yourself or your partner. Never mind that you have a wonderful baby; do some of the clearing exercises in this book *now*, while everything is fresh and fluid, so these feelings won't hang around and haunt you for the next several years. The gamut of feelings can be everything from severe depression or anger about a cesarean you feel was unnecessary to feeling like you made too much noise or should have relaxed more. We would hope by now you're being kinder to yourself, but such feelings and images do sneak in. As midwives we have often been amazed when a woman births with beauty and with power and then apologizes afterwards, as if she didn't "behave properly" or wasn't relaxed enough. VBAC mothers who birth successfully are often hard on themselves because they have set up a list of twenty-five demands, a few of which they didn't achieve. Don't judge yourself yet again for feeling what you feel; allow yourself to experience it and let it go.

The jumble of emotions you feel as a new mother is heightened by the physical changes that are going on in your body. The hormonal change from being pregnant to being a new mother is tremendous, but there are also changes due to interrupted sleep patterns, tiredness, possible anemia, need for vitamins, and so forth. Make sure that you are nourishing yourself with good food and supplements, and nap as often as possible.

A Crisis in Being

It is not so easy for a mother to remember how she related to children before becoming a parent, or how she got to her current state of (relative) ease with children. One of the biggest changes a person must make is obvious if you leave your children with someone who is not a mother. Their greatest area of ineptness will be lapses of consciousness about where the children are, what they are doing, or what they need. A mother (or father, teacher or babysitter who has really acquired these traits) must be aware of the children *at all times*. This is especially true with babies and small children. The sixth sense, "having eyes in the back of your head," or hearing a baby cry from several rooms away are traits that come easiest to the biological mother, but they can be learned by anyone who takes on the life-and-death task. The mother has a psychic link with the baby after it is born, just as she has had a physical link before birth. For example, you are probably alert to your baby's rhythms and may find you wake up seconds before your new baby if you are in the same room. It is virtually impossible for a mother to roll over on a baby while breastfeeding it at night; there's too much connectedness between the two of you.

It is possible for a father to acquire this kind of awareness about the baby, *if* he is willing to undertake the task. But if the two of you decide that he needs to sleep because he has to get up early and go to work in the morning while you can stay home and nap, he will rapidly learn to tune out the baby's cries at night and will become as impervious as a stone. The mother feels she can never be unaware of the baby's needs; at a minimum she can make sure that someone else is handling them, either arranging in advance with someone whom she trusts, or making arrangements or pleas for help each time needs arise.

Making this change to constantly being aware of, and responsible for, a baby is a *big change*. It is a stretch. You suddenly have to take into account someone beside yourself in a way even marriage doesn't demand. (With a toddler you can't even go to the bathroom alone some days!) Feelings of frustration or being overwhelmed are not uncommon as you grow to meet the task. It does get easier. You do increase in your being. And as it becomes easier you become more able to take care of a child and to do other things as well. One of the biggest shocks for first-time mothers is how hard it is to get anything done. We expect too much of ourselves in the first few months. But we also forget that a new mother's entire life is being reorganized. People who have worked all their lives and then stop, whether to have a baby or to retire, often find themselves at a loss without the structure and rhythms that have defined their identity and their waking life in the past. Instead of feeling free and joyous, they don't know what to do, sometimes finding it hard to get out of bed and impossible to accomplish anything. A new mother is in an equally serious state of transition, except that she is in fact *doing* a great deal if she is constantly changing, feeding, and carrying the baby as well as doing the household tasks for herself and the family.

If you can relax and "let it be" for the first six weeks postpartum (the forty days of other cultures), you'll find you will regain your equilibrium. There *is* another side, and you *do* come out on it. Your baby will acquire rhythms of eating and sleeping, you will acquire confidence at diapering and bathing a baby, and you will regain some physical balance as your body settles into being a nursing mother. While it is possible to have an easier postpartum by planning in advance and lining up sufficient help, it is impossible not to go through the inner reorganization required by becoming a first-time mother. If you can accept "business as usual while alterations are in progress" rather than feeling like your life is in a total jumble and will always remain that way, you will make the necessary changes with less discomfort than if you fight them or despair over them.

Rahima once lived communally with a woman who had a baby after months of trying to be aware of children and of what it means to be a mother. She made great progress while living with three children, and she had plenty of positive models in the other adults in the household who had the same ideals. When she had her baby, they all did everything in their power to make the postpartum period as easy as possible for her. She didn't have any of the household responsibilities of a mother in a nuclear family, and there was support with the baby whenever she wanted it. And yet it was not easy for her; she felt stiff and awkward with the newborn and had to go through her own changes in becoming a new mother. One can't be spared the stretch and the growth of motherhood. Were it totally easy, you'd already be there and there would be no growth and no change involved.

A Change for Fathers Too

Going through labor, delivery, and having a new baby is very emotional for a father too, especially if he takes an active part in the birth. If it is a homebirth, he is likely to be thoroughly exhausted once everyone leaves the two of you alone. While he can be of immeasurable help, especially if he is able to be home in the days following the birth, you should arrange for other people to bring casseroles by, etc., to allow him to share with his new family in this wonderful energy and to recover his own bearings.

A father's emotions about his own parents, about being a father, and about responsibility can all weigh heavily on a man—or help to open him up. If he leaves the home to go to work, he steps out of that world and into one of adult conversation and effectiveness; he still needs to maintain an awareness of his wife, how different her physical and psychic state are and how different life is at home. Accepting that everything has changed and will continue to change can be of tremendous help. It is impossible to go back to the way life was before having a baby. And yet the way life seems just after a new baby is not the way it will be in six weeks or six months or two years.

Nourishing Your Relationship as a Couple

If you haven't guessed by now what we're going to say, you must really be in a postpartum muddle. *Communicate with each other.* Share your joys in the new baby. Express your fears and frustrations. If you're having a hard time (and you may not be), at least communicate with each other about it, so you'll feel like you're holding hands and sinking together! You'll also rise together as life takes on its new forms. That's much better than feeling all alone and blaming the other person for not being more supportive or making you feel better.

If you've been communicating throughout pregnancy, you probably won't need the following exercise, but you might want to try it.

The thing that surprised me most about the baby was . . .

_____

_____

_____

The thing that I find most difficult about being a new parent is . . .

_____

_____

_____

The thing I like most about being a new parent is . . .

_____

_____

_____

My partner is being . . .

_____

_____

_____

The thing I wish they had told me about it is . . .

_____

_____

_____

I wish I had . . .

_____

_____

_____

I wish I could . . .

_____

_____

_____

I wish my partner would . . .

_____

_____

_____

List everything you did today:

_____

_____

_____

Tenderness, affection and support can really help at this time. Small kindnesses and considerations can be wonderful for a woman after the birth, and can avoid exaggerating problems out of proportion.

Consideration goes both ways, though, and if you have had a hard day at home with a colicky baby and a whining two-year-old, at least greet your husband and give him a kiss before handing him all the children or falling apart. Little things can make a difference.

Is there sex after birth? The concensus seems to be yes, but not right away. Once the lochial discharge has stopped (within the first few weeks), there is no medical need to avoid having intercourse; your insides have healed and you are not open to infection or other complications. But, while the approximately 300 women interviewed in _Making Love During Pregnancy_ reported varying experiences during the nine months of pregnancy, the overwhelming majority reported difficulty in resuming lovemaking postpartum.[2] The reasons seem to be partly physiological, partly emotional. Many women report a vaginal dryness in the months after the baby is born; this is due to the hormones involved in lactation and the suppression of ovulation with its slippery mucus. Many women also report a decreased sexual drive while they are breastfeeding. Others just find they feel exhausted and are "touched enough" in the course of the day; all they want at night is to sleep.

Especially if a woman has torn or had an episiotomy, she may fear that penetration will be painful. Feeling sexual energy, proceeding with gentleness, and using a lubricant can help in resuming sexual intercourse. Actively taking in your partner's penis and caressing it with your pelvic floor muscles combined with slow and gentle penetration can also be more comfortable than being passive to the event.

Fear of becoming pregnant again right away can also block a woman's sexual response. Although total breastfeeding (without supplements and with night feedings) suppresses ovulation and provides a natural form of family spacing, a woman will ovulate before her first period, and women occasionally ovulate in the first couple of weeks postpartum while their body is adjusting hormonally. Since a nursing mother cannot use the pill and should not use an IUD because her uterus is temporarily porous, a barrier method of birth control can be selected, such as a condom or a diaphragm and spermicidal jelly. Remember that diaphragms should be refitted at six weeks postpartum to make sure you still wear the same size. Charting and natural birth control are more difficult for a nursing mother since she doesn't have regular periods, but couples interested in that method are encouraged to see The Farm's *A Cooperative Method of Natural Birth Control* by Margaret Nofziger.[3]

Sometimes having a baby in the same room can dampen a couple's sexual fervor. Certainly once the baby cries, it is all over. And babies have a tendency to wake during lovemaking, because they are still so connected with the mother's energy. Jeanine Parvati, author of *Hygieia: A Woman's Herbal,*[4] also suggested that they wake up because they don't want another sibling! Could be.

Your sexual life does not need to disappear with the birth of the baby. In fact, continued intimacy and sharing are vital to the health of a marriage. But patience, consideration and give-and-take from both partners are often called for, unless you're so hot for each other you both can't wait. (We know one woman who made love in the hospital on the day she gave birth. Not to be recommended, but hats off!) Things will change. You will heal. Your energy will change. The baby will grow. You will feel sexual again. In the meantime, keep communication open, pleasure each other, avoid resentment and hostility, and remember that this is a time of transition. Women and couples who have children are (or can be) very sexual.

Being with a Newborn

Let us assume for a moment the spiritual view that each person is a very wise and knowing being who comes and inhabits this tiny, growing body to fulfill his or her destiny on earth. That doesn't sound like a very radical view to us, but if it's hard for you to try on, think of it this way. If you knew you were going to be present at the birth of the Messiah or a very great holy person, what would you do? How would you act? What would you feel? Even if you found out later you were wrong, you would have benefited by having elevated yourself to that state of consideration, reverence and concern. And the baby would have benefited by such attendants. So, even if you can't experience the truth of this viewpoint, we ask you to try it on. See whom you like better, the person you are when you think that babies are spiritual beings, or when you think this is the fifth delivery you've done in thirty-six hours and you're already late for your weekend appointment.

Regarding children as coming from an unseen world enables us to be open to sharing in that world when we are around them, for the little children are much closer to the kingdom of heaven than the average adult. This is evidenced very simply in the love and generosity that babies call forth. You'll find with a new baby that everyone stops to talk to you, to adore the baby, to offer you very generous presents, and much more. Babies are love, and they open people's hearts, because people feel that quality when they are around them and forget themselves for the moment.

This viewpoint also allows us to trust in the unfolding development of the child. His or her powers, character and destiny are there in potential from before birth. Certainly they are influenced by yours and your partner's genes and by the parenting and choices you make—but perhaps your child also chooses you. While you must still do your best, you are not the only ones responsible for who your child will be as an adult.

Returning to the image of a very knowing being in a very small body: What's it like being a newborn? There is an obvious disparity between the full power of a spiritual being (who has the potential of working with 25 preschoolers or being President) and that tiny body. The process of full incarnation is a gradual one, with the adult "I" not fully coming in until 21, the age of majority recognized in folk wisdom. In a baby the true self is mostly sleeping, connected with the body and awaking as it develops into its mature capacity to bear with full consciousness the power of soul and spirit functioning through it.

For the baby, the main tasks are taking hold of the body, mastering the process of digestion and bringing the breathing into rhythm. The toddler strives to gain uprightness and the ability to walk and talk, and has its first taste of the "I" between the ages of two and three. The Terrible Twos are really a wonderful time of assertion of the self before it returns to a dreamier state while further development goes on.

Babies are totally identified with each perception or sensation. Think of the process of digestion for your baby. Each bodily sensation, each hunger pang or bubble of air is all-consuming. No reasoning or delay will do any good! In a similar way, when your baby nurses at your breast, the sense of well-being permeates her entire body, causing her eyes to roll up in pure ecstacy.

For the new baby, each sensation is just as consuming. The baby does not have the buffers or filters of an adult that deaden sense impressions. The only way he or she can shut out the world is to go to sleep. Babies sleep so much because they need time to "digest" the impressions that have come to them through the senses.

LeBoyer wrote in *Birth Without Violence* that he attended 3000 births before realizing that the baby's cries and screams at birth were from distress.[5] The knowledge that the newborn is completely sensitive and open is more available to us now. While many people try to make the transition of birth as gentle as possible by having soft lighting, a warm room and no loud noises, consideration for the baby should not stop a few hours after the birth.

Many of us, in reacting against the view that pregnancy is an illness and that babies are fragile, have demonstrated our liberation by strapping the baby in a front carrier and taking him or her everywhere we go, including such places as loud concerts or discount department stores with their crowds and fluorescent lights. Understanding how open a baby is to all these influences might encourage us to consider the quality of the places we go. It may be better for one parent to stay home so the baby can be secure in his own rhythms and familiar space.

It is interesting, too, that many of the traditional ideas of old wives tales that we reject in our efforts to be modern seem to have a deeper wisdom that people have forgotten. For example, in Mexico the people were shocked when Rahima held her baby over her shoulder to burp him. They would never hold a young baby vertically. Rahima showed them that there was no basis to their belief, and certainly Seth seemed none the worse for wear. But in studying about the nervous system and considering the weight of the head and brain in relation to the spinal cord, as well as the subtle centers of psychic energy (chakras) and their relation to the body, one might agree that babies are better left horizontal until they have their own head/neck control and can sit up unsupported.

In a similar way, the fontanelles or "soft spots" on the head are accorded much respect in Mexico. The baby's head is always covered, and the child is protected from direct sunlight. Only *gringos* let their babies go out with nothing on but a diaper while the sun pours down. Those spiritual teachers who have turned their attention to the development of the child speak of the importance of the fontanelles that are open to higher influences, the difference for the child once they have closed, and the power of the sun on children of all ages.

Maintaining the warmth of a baby is also very important. Babies' internal temperature-regulating systems are not fully developed. Babies need physical warmth just as they need the warmth of love and protection. Any outdoorsman knows that you loose a very large proportion of your body heat through your head. This is especially true for the newborn, whose head is proportionately larger than an adult's, and it is even more true at birth when the head is wet. Keeping a baby's head covered by a soft stockinette cap of silk, cotton or wool knit can both maintain body warmth, protect the fontanelles, and shelter the baby from harsh outside influences.

In a similar way, babies and young children need to be dressed warmly, so their body heat stays with them and is not dissipated. In other cultures babies are always covered, either to keep warm or to protect them from the sun. Warmth seems to be very important in assuring that the person's real being can be connected with the body and take up residency.

In considering ways of keeping your baby warm, you might also think about the quality of the fibers that touch his skin. A baby's skin is extremely sensitive to light and temperature, as well as touch. Babies are prone to rashes, and if we think of how uncomfortable *we* feel in some synthetic fabrics that don't breathe, we can imagine what it is like for a baby. Many mothers are going back to using cloth diapers instead of disposables, and they are using wool coverings such as BioBottoms, or wool-knit soakers instead of rubber pants over the diapers. Wool wicks moisture away from the body while letting in air. Very soft wool is not irritating to the skin. Natural fibers such as wool, silk and cotton have the ability to interact with the body's energy in positive or neutral ways, while chemical fibers tend to rob the body of vitality.

The picture we have given is one of a baby being very protected, sheltered in loving arms, natural fibers and warmth. He or she would ideally be kept away from harsh lights and noises such as the stereo or television. We recommend this not only because the baby's senses are completely open, but because the baby's delicate sense organs are still developing. The effect of electronic voices and music on the developing ear of a baby and young child can detract from their later ability to distinguish between live and recorded tone, for example. The effects of emissions from television and computer display terminals on the developing eye is still a matter of debate in medical circles. As parents, we need to protect our babies and children under the age of seven. No other mammal baby stays so dependent and vulnerable for such a long time as the human being. There is a special process of development we human beings need to undergo if we are to realize our full potential. Regarding the first nine months of life in the outside world as a transition following the nine months spent inside the womb is not an unrealistic picture of the baby's need for protection.

We are not saying that babies are fragile creatures who need to be kept in a rarified atmosphere and handled with kid gloves. Enjoy your baby! Play with him or her, massage her, sing to him, spend time outdoors. Don't tiptoe around when she sleeps. Include him in your chores in the home. But be sensitive to your baby's reactions to strangers, strange places, noises, or long trips.

Creating Rhythm

One of the most disorienting parts of the first few weeks after a baby is born is that there seems to be no rhythm to life. You don't know when your baby will cry or want to nurse or be asleep. You can't plan anything. And your own sleep is often interrupted and irregular. Rhythm in daily life sustains us, and a conscious awareness of rhythm can be a tremendous help toward creating a sense of well-being.

One of the tasks of a newborn is to come into rhythm. Its breathing is irregular, as any mother will attest who has heard her newborn seem to stop breathing, then gasp several times, then breathe normally for a while. One of the things that happens during childhood is that the baby's rapid and irregular heartbeat and breathing patterns gradually assume the rhythm of four heartbeats to each breath that characterize an adult's.

Coming into the rhythm of earthly life is a gradual process, one that begins in infancy. Reacting against the regimen of bottle feeding every four hours regardless of how long a baby cried, most mothers who are breastfeeding have resorted to nursing on demand. The convenience of nursing also lends itself to instantly satisfying your baby's needs, whether physical or emotional, without having to wait for formula to be prepared or for a bottle to be warmed. While we are in no way suggesting that a baby should be left to cry or that adherence to a clock should come between you and your baby, we are suggesting that being aware of creating rhythm while breastfeeding can go a long way toward helping it emerge. For example, holding and rocking a

fussy baby instead of immediately offering the breast may help your baby to respond to other ways of being comforted and to eat when hungry rather than all the time. While a newborn is not to be denied, having an awareness of rhythm will help you recognize patterns as they emerge and will contribute to both your baby's and your own sense of well-being.

Very few breastfed babies sleep through the night, but if you tuck your baby in with you and maintain an aura of sleepiness, your baby will usually fall back to sleep. This is especially true early in the morning. If you greet your several-month-old baby, she will be wide awake and ready to play. But if you maintain a heavy-lidded somnolence, she will nurse and join you for another hour or two of needed sleep.

Be sensitive to your baby. Take your cues from him or her. Get to know her cries, her patterns, her new gestures and movements as they appear. Trust yourself, trust your partner, trust your ability to learn and to respond to the needs of this new being. It won't take long before you are experienced at recognizing your baby's various cries and other ways of communicating. Being with a newborn is a wonderful experience—don't miss the opportunity to just *be* together. Babies are big on being and small on doing. Be with him or her, and enjoy.

Fathering and Mothering

Many couples today have welcomed the man's assuming a more nurturing role with the children. Nurturing children involves more being and awareness than doing. It is not goal-oriented, and very little seems to get accomplished. As men have come to honor this work and to develop the nurturing aspect of themselves, they sometimes ask if there is really a difference between the father's presence and the mother's. Women also sometimes ask about the nature of biological mothering compared with fathering, or the mothering that another woman might consciously undertake for a child not biologically hers.

Rahima is going to make a controversial statement that there is a unique relationship between the biological mother and her baby during the first months and years of life, just as there was during pregnancy. Up to the age of three years there is an invisible bond with the mother that protects and nourishes the child and that deserves honoring by supporting the mother and child being together.

With regard to a young baby, people will sometimes say, "Yes, of course there's breastfeeding, but other than that . . ." Not only must breastfeeding not be discounted, for it provides a unique kind of nourishment that goes beyond anything chemists can copy, but there is also more going on than meets the eye during the first three years. Some time between the ages of 3 and 3½ there is usually a noticeable freeing from the mother. This new independence makes it a better time for beginning preschool than age 2½ or "potty-trained." But keeping your child home is of equal or greater value than preschool. If you and your child are both happy, there is plenty of time later for socializing with peers.

Sometimes fathers, aware of the unique bond between mother and baby, may be jealous of it if they want to be "important to the baby too." Certainly fathers are vital to the life and nurturing of the child, but in a way different from the mother's when the child is very young. This should not be interpreted to mean that therefore both men and women aren't equally capable of changing diapers or that child-rearing and discipline are the mother's exclusive responsibility. Mothers should also not become so caught up in the baby that they don't allow the father to form his own unique relationship with the child. Especially those men who are involved in the pregnancy and birth of their babies often show a tremendous closeness with their children, even when they are quite little, and this needs to be given space in which to grow.

While a man has a developing relationship with the child, and a direct relationship with his wife as a marriage partner, he also has a new relationship with her as a mother. A desire to provide for and protect his family is not chauvinistic; it supports the woman in her mothering. Obviously a single mother can raise a child on her own, but if a woman feels supported both physically and emotionally, she more easily has the psychic strength required for mothering. Encouragement of the mother with a baby can grow into supporting her in different ways with an older child, which we discuss in the next chapter.

Discuss some of these ideas with your partner. Where do you agree or disagree with us? With each other? Discovering the questions of parenting is the task at hand. The answers require the test of living.

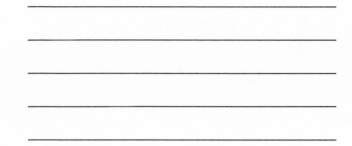

Resources in Case of Complications

The most frequent questions new parents have are: "Is my baby all right?" "Is he or she normal?" "Is *this* normal?" Arrange in advance for a pediatrician to check your baby after the birth. Such an exam is required before you are released from the hospital. For a homebirth, your midwife will probably do a newborn exam but will also recommend that you see a pediatrician or have one lined up ahead of time.

Pick a pediatrician who is compatible with your views of medicine and mothering. Find one who actively supports breastfeeding and who values parents and babies being together. Talk to your friends, childbirth educators or La Leche League leaders to find such a doctor. Arrange in advance for him or her to check the baby after the birth, preferably in your presence. Having a doctor with whom you can work can make a tremendous difference if complications should arise.

A couple in Colorado gave birth at home to a baby who was under five pounds. They took "potluck" in calling a pediatrician to have the baby checked. He said because of the baby's weight it needed to be in the hospital. When they declined, he threatened to charge them with child abuse. What could they do?

They found another pediatrician, called the first to say they dismissed him and advised him they were now working with the other doctor. This second doctor was willing to look at the baby's individual situation, had her brought to the office for blood-sugar tests, and determined that she was full-term and fine without separating the family through hospitalization. Knowing this doctor ahead of time would have saved this couple tremendous anguish.

While you are being reassured by your doctor and midwife that your baby is normal, ask lots of questions so that the unknown won't continue to worry you. Examine your baby yourself—take his or her diaper off and check from head to foot. (A typical newborn exam is outlined in *Special Delivery*.)

What if something abnormal appears? The most common cause of concern is physiological jaundice in days 3 to 7. Your baby will appear yellow-orange if the liver is having trouble breaking down the extra red blood cells that are no longer needed once the baby breathes air. Understanding the facts about the condition, its expected course and possible dangers helps you to make informed decisions. Such information is outlined in *Special Delivery* or is available from your health-care provider. Remember that physicians and hospitals vary greatly in the treatments they recommend; some begin phototherapy at a bilirubin level of 10 while others wait until 20. In addition to breastfeeding and putting your baby in sunlight to help lower the bilirubin level, you can now frequently find support for setting up bili lights at home so your baby doesn't have to enter the hospital.

Remember, in any situation involving your baby's health, you always have choices, probably more than have occurred to you. Hopefully your doctor will suggest various courses of action while leaving the choice up to you. And you can always ask for a second medical opinion from a doctor not in his medical group. You can change doctors if necessary, including trying an alternative health professional such as a naturopathic physician. When confronting an array of medical tests, a helpful question can be, "What are the results of this test going to do for us, i.e. how will knowing affect the course of treatment or our decisions?" If the treatment is the same in either case, maybe the test isn't necessary.

Do parents have the legal right to determine medical treatment for their child? Numerous legal actions and instances of the child being declared a ward of the court while the parents are charged with negligence or abuse make this a difficult question to answer positively. It is worthwhile to find a physician with whom you can work before complications occur. If your baby is sick, you need to have the sense that you are working together, not at cross purposes.

If your baby requires hospitalization for any reason, from prematurity to congenital abnormalities or a neonatal disease, try to be with the baby as much as possible. Your presence and touch even through the portals of an isolette, and your breast-milk can make a tremendous difference in your baby's chance of recovery and your own emotional state. Commitment to the baby, to opening and loving and being involved with that child, really help call the baby to life on this earth. Or it can make letting go more possible should your baby decide not to join ordinary life with you. Arrange to get help expressing your milk—contact the hospital's milk bank or La Leche League for help in learning to use a breast pump if your baby is not allowed to nurse. Breastmilk contains a factor that helps premature babies gain weight; insist on it! Expressing your milk also helps you to keep up your milk supply so you can nurse the baby when it comes home.

Any kind of physical abnormality involves all of the emotions of grieving. Anger, blame, bargaining, guilt, depression—all of these may follow. You are grieving your baby's loss of health and perfection and the loss of your own dreams as well as the difficulties of the situation in which you find yourselves. Seek help in expressing your emotions with your childbirth educator, friend or counselor. Remember to allow yourself and your partner your own ways of grieving, of expressing it or not, and of dealing with the business at hand. Having a child with a birth defect is a great strain on a marriage. If you feel you are sinking, try to hold together as a couple so that, as you are coming back up, it becomes something you have lived through together in your marriage, rather than something that has come between you.

If your child is stillborn or is not expected to live, you can ask to see and hold the baby. Many hospitals understand bonding and grieving in the wake of work done by Klaus and others, and they will be supportive of things that help the parents. But other hospitals still want to whisk the baby away, to "spare you the pain." But the reality of the baby is never as bad as your imagination, and the ability to hold and talk to the baby, to name him or her, to express your feelings and to say "goodbye" can all help tremendously in the healing process. They keep you from becoming stuck in denial and give your aching arms something to hold while you say goodbye. It is also recommended that you request the baby's body for burial or cremation and that you have a funeral or create your own memorial service. Ceremony allows for the expression, sharing and working through of our feelings within the context of community, and can be a valuable element in the healing process.

If you must stay in the hospital after the loss of a baby, request that your room be on a different floor than the newborn nursery or maternity ward if the hospital has not had the courtesy to think of that. If you have birthed at home, you will need to notify a physician and the coroner of the death of the child if you are not already underway to a hospital.

Many communities have support groups for families that have lost a baby. Contact your local childbirth educators or hospice groups to see if one exists in your area. Read *Ended Beginnings* by Panuthos and Romeo.[6] Allow yourself time to grieve. Allow your partner to do so in his way. And don't forget that your other children also need special attention, because they sometimes feel that their jealousy or not wanting a new baby has killed the child. Healing takes time. If this happens to you, you will move through it, but it won't go away. You will always remember this child, this birth and death, this loss and all that you will gain through it in understanding, strength and compassion.

Help with Breastfeeding

Many times a baby is perfectly healthy, but complications develop with breastfeeding. If the baby won't nurse or if you develop a breast infection, you need advice that will lead to successful nursing, not to bottle feeding and weaning. Making contact with La Leche League during your pregnancy by attending their monthly meetings and having the number of their telephone counseling line is invaluable insurance. League leaders are knowledgeable, trained and dedicated to helping you succeed, whether the difficulties are minor or major. Many doctors do not have information as accurate as the League's. It's good to know they are as close as your telephone.

The Choices Don't Go Away

Just as you had to inform yourself to create the kind of birth experience you wanted for your baby, you will find that the questions and issues of parenting involve a similar process of finding out the facts, weighing your own reactions and values, and making the best decisions you can, ones for which you will have to take responsibility as you live with them. Even if your child is completely healthy, as most children are, you will have decisions about circumcision, immunizations, childcare, education, and on and on. You can never fully know what the outcome will be. Don't do things solely for the future, like making your baby's birth as gentle as possible or doing a "LeBoyer bath" so he or she will be even-tempered and ambidextrous! Do them only if it feels like the most aware, responsible and furthering thing to do in the moment, because you have no guarantees how your child will grow up. Your children have their own destinies, their own difficulties to overcome or to live with. You and your choices are not the sole determinants of the way they turn out. This does not absolve you of responsibility, but your responsibility is simply to do the best you can—which of course you do. As you evolve and grow throughout your parenting life, you will see that, were you to do things over again, knowing what you know now, you would probably choose to do things differently. But given who you were then and what you knew and the way things were, you made the best decisions you could, just as your own parents did with you. In becoming parents we join, sometimes consciously, sometimes unconsciously, in the unfoldment of the human race on this planet from one generation to the next. *L'chaim!* (Hebrew: "To Life!")

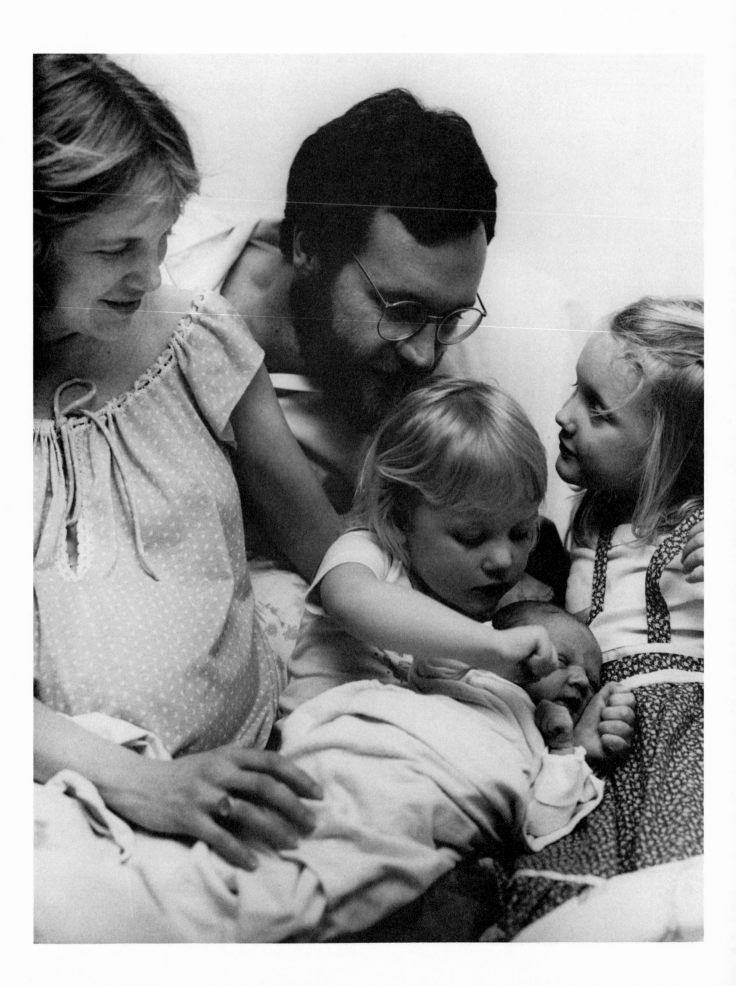

12
For Not-So-New Parents

If you have older children, you have probably already experienced some of the pitfalls described here. For those of you having your first child, we hope the following will help you traverse the path through parenthood without some of the same detours.

Many of these ideas as well as a wealth of other suggestions are developed in greater detail in Rahima's book *You Are Your Child's First Teacher,* which discusses child development and parenting from birth through age six. The book draws from the work of Austrian educator Rudolf Steiner as well as contemporary child development specialists and her own experiences as a mother and Waldorf early childhood teacher.

Most people today don't leave a newborn to cry it out or think that a baby is being fussy just to annoy them. But at what stage do we start thinking, as Lewis Carroll said, "He only does it to annoy,/For he can thoroughly enjoy/The pepper when he pleases"? Usually after the age of two parents start to feel that their child has acquired some "negative" traits like selfishness, stubborness, a temper, irrationality, or a whiney or manipulative way. The most common reaction is to blame oneself. This is not only a typical reaction for a woman, but it is strengthened by the fact that we are probably seeing characteristics that we don't like in ourselves. Otherwise we wouldn't react so strongly to them in our children.

In fact what is happening is the first real assertion of the "I" between ages two and three, which we discussed in the last chapter. Understanding can help us to meet with more equanimity a child who is particularly powerful, realizing that we must correct him and provide examples of right action over and over again, and do it without our own emotional reactions.

With a first child it is difficult to gain perspective because few parents have a comprehensive overview of child development and they don't have another child with whom to compare. It took Rahima's having a second child to realize that her mothering must be all right if there could be two so completely opposite mirrors of it. For example, her second child would wake up all sweetness and light, "Oh, I love you, Mommy!" The first would wake up with the same argument with which he had gone to bed.

What Rahima was seeing is an example of the difference in temperaments that children and adults manifest. Temperaments can be understood as groups of traits that dominate in different people. Some children are very powerful, with tremendous force of will and action. They tend to dominate in play, using images of power such as eagles, tornados or bears. In boys of this type, there tends to be anger and aggression that they just can't control. They can be very overbearing, but have positive leadership ability. They tend to be compactly and powerfully built, and walk with their heels dug into the ground. A classic example in adult life would be Napoleon.

Contrast that child with one who is very dreamy and likes to sit. Sometimes movement seems like too much effort for this type of child. These children are very involved in the comfort of their bodies, and their favorite part of the day will be snack time. When they interact with other children, they usually have a harmonizing effect; more often they are content to just sit and watch. This type of child is very different from the first one described! These two children will present very different challenges to their parents and teachers, because they learn differently and need to be taught differently.

A third type of temperament is the child who is almost always bright and happy. He or she is usually very cheerful, with tears changing to laughter as quickly as they appear. This child seems to barely touch the ground, and in fact can be observed to walk on the toes much of the time. These children can be very easy to parent; the difficulty in the elementary grades is that their interest is so ephemeral

that they're like a butterfly flitting from one thing to the next. Depth and seeing a project through to completion are difficult for this type of child.

To round out our description of the temperaments, picture a child who is often very inward, more involved in his or her own emotional world than in external action. This kind of child is not so easy to spot in early childhood, because most young children seem to be happy much of the time. But as they grow older they seem to take everything personally, bearing a great deal of suffering (because someone doesn't like him, or because one child didn't give her a Valentine). Crying at his or her birthday party is often typical of this child. The positive side of this temperament is a very compassionate and caring nature.

The study of temperaments can be very helpful for parenting, teaching, or work on oneself in becoming more balanced. What we have given is only the briefest of descriptions, but it should reassure you that children are different from one another and from their parents.[1] They require special understanding if their needs are to be met. It is sometimes most difficult when a mother and child have opposite temperaments or when they have the same temperament and the mother isn't reconciled to those qualities in herself.

Underline the words that most describe your child (or yourself if you have no child over the age of three). Obviously your child will manifest all of these at some time, but pick the ones that you see most often.

outgoing	willful	fearless
friendly	sensitive	kind
shy	happy	comfortable
cautious	active	dependent
angry	quiet	independent
whiney	powerful	inward
easy	passive	tolerant
stubborn		

(fill in more words)

_____

_____

_____

Put a (+) by characteristics you like; a (−) by those you don't like. How many of them do you share with your child?

"You're Not the Boss of Me"

This frequent remark of Rahima's son from the age of two to five called into question a common dilemma of parents today. What is the relationship of parents to their children? What kind of authority do parents have, and how do they want to manifest it? Such a question would have been unthinkable fifty or a hundred years ago, but today many parents don't want to appear authoritarian and are searching for new forms to express what is needed. While it seems contradictory to many people to spank a child while saying, "Don't hit," the opposite extreme of not doing anything until you explode in overreaction is equally unproductive.

It is necessary—and possible—that children behave. They need to assume the social values of sharing and using their words instead of their fists. But they also can be expected to do as they are told and not to talk back or reason you into a corner. In an effort today to be fair and/or be pals with their children, parents spend endless amounts of time reasoning with their preschoolers or letting them run roughshod over their lives. But how can you get compliance?

Children under the age of seven really don't have the type of memory necessary to recall what they did or to have a punishment deter them from doing it the next time. That type of memory first starts appearing at age five, when it is *possible* to achieve an effect from saying "Remember . . ." or "You *should* . . ." Prior to the age of five, children learn almost entirely through imitation and repetition. They have "body memory" and memory that is triggered by sense impressions, but they can't call something up at will. Abstract thought has little effect on their behavior.

If you want a young child to do something, it is most effective to do it with him or her. Using a positive statement like, "We do it this way" while you do it in front of or with the child will get her actually doing it without the problems engendered by, "Eat with your spoon" or, "Clean up your toys." Children can't help but imitate the movements of the people around them. This demands that adults, who are notoriously sedentary, get up off their bums and do something with a child. But the cooperation, harmony and learning that are accomplished are far more effective than commands, threats or promises.

As another example, you can tell a five-year-old a hundred times not to slam the screen door, and it will have no effect. But if you gather your intention, meet the child at the door and close the door gently with his hand, saying firmly, "We close the door quietly," the lesson will probably get through.

In addition to imitation, fantasy can be used to accomplish what you want without resistance. Making something into a game or adding just the tiniest wisp of imagination can make "going upstairs to nap as quietly as little mice" or having the "moving men" put away all the blocks difficult to resist. Similarly, if children are playing train right across the walkway, entering into their imagination and asking the engineers to move the chairs while you start to do it with them will work more effectively than asking them wouldn't they like to move their train or asking them to break their imagination and become children who are in the way.

A great many discipline problems can be avoided if parents have the conviction that they can both insist on right action and that they can't expect the preschooler to remember it. What is involved is a more or less constant repetition of doing it the right way with the child. Over time you will see improvement, both as those new habit patterns work their way into the body and as the child matures. It is usually our annoyance or feeling of powerlessness in the face of a child who does something for the hundredth time that is our downfall. Understanding the young child can help us to keep perspective on his or her behavior.

Parents also need to support each other. It is especially important that the father supports the mother by taking the same kind of correcting action with the child when both parents are in the room (rather than always letting her do it) and by backing up the mother with statements like, "Listen to your mother" or "Don't talk to her like that." This tells the child that the parents are united and that it is impossible to pit one against the other.

If you are not getting that kind of support from your husband, ask him about it. Do you have differing views that have never been expressed? Is he oblivious to what is going on? What do you need to feel supported? What does your child need?

_____

_____

_____

Rhythm to the Rescue

Establishing rhythm and developing repeating rituals can go a long way toward making your child feel secure and avoiding discipline problems. Anyone who has had to read the same bedtime story to a child every night for three months knows how much children are nourished by things staying the same. If you get your hair cut or wear your husband's sweater you may notice your two- or three-year-old being very upset. This is because their sense of well-being is related to the security of things being the same.

Daily rhythm can be especially helpful at meal times and at nap and bedtimes. The fact that these events occur regularly, at the same time and in the same way, without discussion and without fail, makes life so much simpler for both the children and the adults. Many parents think that because they have difficulty putting their child to bed, they should therefore let her stay up until their bedtime. Young children need eleven or twelve hours of sleep or rest each night—even the wide-awake ones. If you are putting your two-year-old to bed at 10 p.m., that is certainly your choice, but you could be starting your bedtime ritual at 7 or 7:30 and the child would sleep that extra time, without complaint. And you would have some evening left for adult activities and conversation. What it takes to establish a rhythm is unlimited intention that it is going to work and about three days for the child to adjust. Children need rest and sleep as a time in which to digest all of the impressions of the day. But they love consciousness and cling to it, so only a child who is used to a set rhythm will ask to be put to bed.

Bedtime can be helped by quiet play after dinner and a definite bedtime ritual, which involves getting ready for bed before quiet time together (usually a story or songs), and then sleep. Most people read to their children, but telling stories that you have read or made up or which are just simple incidents from your own childhood is really appreciated by children. Fairy tales are also especially nourishing to young children because they depict the inner soul/spiritual world from which the child has so recently come. All of the characters in a fairy tale are contained within each person. If you read or tell a fairy tale, do so in a melodic, rhythmical voice as if you are narrating events that happened in another world. Avoid changing your voice and dramatizing the parts; that way the justice and violence in a fairy tale will not upset your child but will lead to appropriate resolution, which the fairy tale always contains.

Singing can also be a wonderful part of bedtime. There is a simple instrument called a "Children's Harp" which is specially tuned in the pentatonic scale so that anyone can make beautiful music on it.[2] It is a wonderful way to lull your child into the nourishing world of sleep. Many parents also like to light a candle while they are telling a story to their child. The candle light is very soft, and watching a candle flame can help to calm a very active child. Be sure to light the candle with great ceremony and perhaps with a song, and blow it out (or let the child do so) before you leave the room.

Think of sleep as a time of physical and spiritual renewal. How does your child go off to sleep? Is there a regular time and a regular ritual? Write down what you do now:

_____

_____

_____

If you would like to change anything, write down what you would like to see happen. Talk it over with your partner, and begin tonight!

_____

_____

_____

Mealtime can also be enriched by a candle, a permanent place where each person sits, a blessing that is said or sung, and flowers or placemats on the table. If a child whines or complains during dinner, he or she can be taken out. With young children it is necessary to go with them, rather than sending them out. But if you are stern, don't give them special attention when out, and tell them that as soon as they are a "happy clown" or have a "happy face" they can return to the group, they will straighten up within two minutes. This simple action of removal and return can avert endless bantering, cajoling and eventual loss of temper. Keeping in mind that young children live so much in the realm of gesture and action, the movement will speak to them much more directly than reasoning, pleading or threatening.

Rhythm can also be applied to the days of the week and the seasons of the year. Long ago life had a natural rhythm—Monday was wash day, Tuesday was baking day, Thursday was ironing day, and so forth. As busy as most of us are, we are lucky when anything gets done, let alone regularly; most people do not even observe the Sabbath as a day apart from any of the others in the week. To the extent that we can give rhythm to our children, they will acquire a sense of the day and of the week. Going to the park regularly, or doing a crafts project together on a certain day each week, or going to story time at the library once a week help a child to understand the succession and rhythm of the week.

A similar attention to the seasons and the festivals of the year can help maintain an awareness of the aliveness of nature and the cyclical character of the course of the year. Children love the festive preparations for a holiday—baking, singing, making the same decorations each year. These are ways in which we can provide a framework for their growing and changing lives.

"Let's Talk About It"

Many parents who have discovered the damage that repressing emotions has caused in their own lives, fall into the trap of wanting their children to express all their emotions fully. While we are not advocating repressing emotion, the current trend to make children aware of and express everything they feel has unexpected side effects. These children become very awake emotionally and very manipulative, especially with their parents.

Young children are totally open to their physical and emotional surroundings, but they lack the inner emotional complexity of an adolescent or an adult. For the young child, most emotions are like ripples on a lake—they pass quickly and don't penetrate very deeply into consciousness. This is why tears can change to laughter through a kiss or a small diversion of attention. If a young child is frightened or angry, the upset needs to be handled in the present moment with a hug, a few words or whatever will help the child regain equilibrium. But then the emotion is past and, for the most part, forgotten unless the parents bring it up again for analysis.

Young children do not have the same kind of memory as adults. That is why a fight with your child on the way to preschool can leave you in a bad mood all morning, but he or she is happy moments after leaving you. The extent to which

adults carry the past and want to analyze everything with a young child is frequently illustrated in Rahima's preschool when a mother or father picks up the child at 5 p.m. and wants to discuss the situation of eight o'clock that morning. Nothing could be further from the child's reality! But the child who has become used to such "discussions" will dredge up something suitable for the parents, for this is one of their primary ways of interacting.

Most parents are too analytical and rational with their preschoolers, producing a self-awareness that is inappropriate and even unhealthy in a child under seven. We have even seen parents make preschoolers "practice" different emotional situations and responses. This kind of emotional work, suitable perhaps for an adult doing inner work, is way beyond the emotional development of a young child. As a result the child not only becomes very conscious of his or her emotions, but begins to notice the effects they can have on other people. Such children feel that every little thing is terribly important, expecting the same amount of attention the parent gives. Histrionics over small issues and using emotions to get their own way are common when so much attention has been placed on what the child is feeling. Young children's emotions are best acknowledged and allowed to change, not dwelt on.

"Play with Me, Mommy!"

It is amazing the number of children who have forgotten how to play. Left to their own devices, they are at a loss and require constant adult input and involvement. Parents, on the other hand, have bought into the idea of quality time to make up for all the time they aren't with their children, but they find that doing puzzles together for half an hour feels artificial or isn't satisfying to either party.

A first step toward creating a more integrated life is to let the children do more things with you. Children love to "help," to be doing the same things an adult is doing if they aren't forced to do so. So let your child fold the laundry with you or hold the dustpan or help with the dishes. It will take you longer, but the time you spend together will be shared and will be a delight for your child.

It is beneficial for children to see adults doing real work—their fascination with construction sights or workmen is universal. When they can see things being transformed through our hands, they see the human element at its best in a person's ability to be creative. So much of our work has been taken away from us today—perhaps some children see their mothers bake bread, but very few get to watch or imitate ironing. What do our children see us doing most, Rahima asks as she pounds away at the typewriter? Providing examples of work, with real movement and examples they can imitate in their play, enables children to try on the roles and actions of adult life.

Children take everything into their being and will imitate not only the actions they see, but also the emotions behind them. For example, if they see a workman hammering in anger, they will copy the entire gesture in their play, not just quietly hammer on something. For this reason it is good to watch the quality of our gestures around a young child. Do we fling something aside in carelessness or anger? Do we stir the cake batter much too fast when our four-year-old is there? Our attention to detail and movement can really help the development of the young child.

Aside from providing children with chances to observe and help with real work, we can provide them with toys that let them transform life into their play. Child-sized brooms, hammers, dishes, and so forth, lend themselves to imaginative play. And toys of natural materials, such as wood, cotton or wool, connect the child to something living.

Toys that are unfinished or archetypal lend themselves to imaginative play more than the plastic figures that are completely finished. A simple stand-up doll made of felt and stuffed with wool can be any of several characters, whereas a Star Wars figure has a definite and fixed identity and mode of action. Simple knot dolls made without faces enable the child to have that doll be a boy or a girl, and be happy, sad or angry. This is in marked contrast to the chrome and plastic dolls with their painted faces or imbecilic expressions.³

Children want to grow and finish their own bodies. By having to finish the dolls and toys with their imaginations, they are involved in the real work of early childhood. Such simple toys as a pine cone and a chunk of wood that has been whittled a bit lend themselves to the imaginative transformations children naturally bring forth. First it is a boat, then a person, then a log under which treasure is hidden. Given a few simple toys and a few simple costumes, children can be happy for hours playing by themselves or with one another.

Another reason that many children can't play is that they have become passive from always having adults do something for them and from watching so much television. The average preschool child watches six hours of television a day, time when the child is unnaturally motionless while being bombarded by images. A child used to creative play will ignore television or will want to turn off "Sesame Street" so she can play with her own puppets (imitation). But children who have been brought up on television as a before-dinner and Saturday-morning babysitter will sit passively or will only imitate the kinds of purposeless movement they see on the screen or in the cartoon characters.

Television also decreases the child's imaginative powers by providing powerful images that go in and come right back out in imitative movement. Stories which are heard, on the other hand, demand the child make them his or her own before acting them out in free play. The difference in the play of preschool and kindergarten children who have watched television or who have not is very noticeable.

If children are allowed time and space to play on their own, a progression in their imaginative play will become apparent. Play for the child under three years primarily involves large movement and getting control of the body—jumping, running, climbing. Around the age of 2½ to 3, the imaginative element will start to enter into play, but play will be primarily solitary. Several children of that age will play next to each other but not really together. By the age of four social interaction is predominate in group imaginative play, and by age 5 they are likely to spend more time planning who will be what than actually doing the scene. Play has the valuable role of helping the child come into earthly life, and internalize the impressions taken in. Children are a real mirror in their play for the gestures and tone of voice of their parents, siblings, teachers and television—in short, everything that they perceive works very deeply and will be expressed in their play.

The dilemma of the first child is that there is usually too much adult attention and concern. Such children tend to be overprotected and become overachievers because they have had all of their parents' time and anxiety showered upon them. With second and third children, the mother is more relaxed, and doesn't have the time she had with a first child. If there are no other children in the neighborhood, or if the child remains an only child, a conscious effort can be made to have children over or to arrange an informal play group or participate in a nursery school. Children need the time to play alone and with other children in an environment that encourages creative play; otherwise they are being robbed of an important part of their childhood.

"When You Are Older . . ."

Parents today often fail to realize that there is any difference between younger and older children. In an effort to be fair they may take all of their children to the same movie, or they may let the three-year-old play video games like Dad or an older brother. Young children not only have a different consciousness, memory, relationship to space and time, and ability to reason than an adult or an older child, but they also have a greater need for protection of their senses than an older brother or sister. Although a child is born with all his or her organs present, part of the process of development in the first seven years is the further growth and differentiation of these organs on the physical level and a less tangible transformation of them as the child's own being refashions what heredity has given and makes it her or his own.[4] During this time of rapid growth and transformation in the first seven years, all of the impressions a child takes in work on his sense organs and inner organs, determining their health and ability throughout later life. For this reason a computer terminal does not have the same effect on a child of twelve as on a child of three. The child under the age of seven is completely imitative—he can't help taking everything in, letting it work on him, and acting it out again. The older child has already outgrown that stage of physical development, has a more developed emotional sphere and awakening powers of critical reason that are coming to the fore.

Most people are aware today of the importance of crawling. Children who have skipped that stage due to leg casts or other medical reasons often experience lack of coordination as an adult and even notice effects in their thinking and emotions. Hours are spent working with such adults and with impaired children in what is called *patterning* (moving their limbs through the endless repetitions of cross crawling). As this kind of work becomes more widely known, it is hoped that parents won't put their babies in baby walkers, which keep them vertical when they should be crawling. They may be convenient, but it is one of many ways in which we try to help our children be in stages they haven't yet reached on their own.

In a similar way, it is possible but unadvisable to speed up development in early childhood by teaching a child to read and write when he is three or four years old. Advertisements to "build a better baby" prey upon parents' anxiety and spiritual materialism by getting them to try teaching their nine-month-old to read by taking an expensive course and using flash cards. Many children can be taught reading and math at an early age; others only start to feel like failures. But success has its price, for this premature awakening of the intellect robs the child of other imaginative powers that form the wellspring for much creativity later in life. The predominance of the imagination that is every young child's birthright begins to fade of its own accord around the age of six or seven and is replaced by an emotional and artistic approach to the world; the puppet shows that still work with a five-year-old will not work in the same way with an eight-year-old, due to the natural growing out of the magical world in which the young child lives. Hastening this growing up process robs the child of vitality and can result in an early loss of roundness of the body characteristic of a young child as well as premature aging of the emotions. Few things are as bad as a jaded five-year-old!

Allowing the child to stay in this magical world of early childhood is not detrimental to his or her cognitive development. On the contrary, the movement games and fingerplays of early childhood help the brain to develop, and the free transformation of objects in creative play is appropriate preparation for the manipulation of symbols involved in reading.

Most children today learn to write their names and other letters almost by osmosis. It is so prevalent in the home through television, older brothers and sisters or parental encouragement. A natural interest in reading and writing should always be encouraged, but the practice of formally teaching the child or making kindergartners spend hours at desks doing unimaginative workbooks is an affront to early childhood. Preschools and kindergartens have changed drastically in the past thirty years as everything has been pushed earlier and earlier; the fact that up to 50 percent of children in some areas are *failing* kindergarten is met with programs for still younger children rather than recognizing that children need to play until their maturity, hand-eye coordination and total consciousness have reached the level of a six- or seven-year-old.

Children who wait until six or seven before beginning book work experience no difficulty in catching up with and excelling over children who have had years of reading or reading-readiness exercises. They are so ready and so eager, that they usually take to it without difficulty. Reading really involves a decoding process. Once the light goes on and the child has discovered the key, he takes off; until that time he needs to be kept from feeling like a failure.

Children who show a natural interest in reading and writing at age five can just be applauded and told that "soon" they will be able to learn to read. Parents need not feel anxiety that this is the critical period that must be seized or lost. Anticipation is a positive force in education. Rahima's oldest children both have November birthdays, and both are very bright. With her first child she emphasized early learning and had him in a highly structured preschool program that taught him to read by age four. By age six he was like a forty-year-old midget, outraged at being in such a small and impotent body that had to be excluded from adult conversations, go to bed before adults, and so forth. When he came into a Waldorf (Rudolf Steiner) school in grade 2, he became much younger, much more emotionally and artistically balanced, and much happier being a child.

Rahima's second child started in a Waldorf kindergarten, which emphasized creative play and the principles described above. Rahima even decided to keep her in the kindergarten a second year because her birthday was in the fall. She had a wonderful extra year of play, and only three times did she "wake up" and ask, "Why aren't I in first grade?" But she never stayed awake long enough for an answer (like the time she said, "You're really Santa Claus aren't you?", but she went away before any answer could be given). She thus was kept away from reading until the end of first grade (age 7½). By the following September she was reading well above second grade level and in third grade was reading *Little Women,* all twelve Oz books and everything she could get her hands on.

Parents have such an anxiety that their children won't learn fast enough—whether it is to walk or be toilet trained or read. They are afraid they won't get into the right colleges, schools and even preschools! Children unfold according to their own timetable, and allowing that to happen without pushing is important for balanced development. This is a plea for parents to relax and let their children be children. If you need more eloquent or more detailed argu-

ments, see *The Hurried Child* by David Elkind[5] or *School Can Wait* and *Better Late than Early* by Raymond and Dorothy Moore.[6]

Maintaining the Unity

The world surrounding a young child should be an expression of the unity which the child feels. The baby can only gradually differentiate itself from its mother or other surroundings. The baby is the center of its own universe, or one can say that there is no sense of inside and outside. That world gradually changes as the baby discovers her hands and then learns to sit, to crawl and to walk. But the child is still in a unitive world, and assumes that everything is good and worthy of imitation. It experiences everything with its senses and its entire body and puts it into movement. The discriminating power of the intellect is still slumbering in the young child. A premature emphasis on reading, writing and reasoning can bring too much consciousness too soon in the intellectual sphere, with its predominance of analysis and picking things apart. The unity becomes shattered.

Too much consciousness of the emotions also leads to premature self awareness and manipulative behavior rather than emotions being fluid ripples on the surface of the water as they are for a young child. Similarly, the current emphasis on vitamins, nutrition and allergies is making three-year-olds overly conscious of everything they eat, dissecting it first and doubting its goodness. Parents need to be aware of nutrition for their child, but a young child is better left without the details.

Assuming the spiritual view that children are involved in a process of incarnation that occurs gradually over time, what young children need is for their parents to surround them with a world of warmth and love that is unitive and good, in which they need not be too aware of the finer points of abstract logic or minimum daily requirements. The circle game expresses this unitive picture of early childhood and the "falling down" process of coming into earthly life. Children delight in the circle and in the falling down, as long as they don't hit too hard. Circle games are favorites of young children, but children don't usually want to be singled out to be the main character until around the age of five. Being the "farmer" or the "cheese" usually involves more self-consciousness than most three-year-olds are ready to handle.

How can we respect this unitive picture of the world that young children have and allow their coming into earthly life to be a gentle transition from the spiritual world? The answers to that question go beyond the scope of this book. But a Waldorf preschool which takes that question seriously in determining both the environment and the activities is very different from a preschool in which the goal is to make everything as conscious as possible. If you are interested in more information, you can refer to Rahima's article on "The Magical Years, Some Waldorf Indications for Early Childhood" in *Mothering Magazine*.[7] Waldorf schools were first founded by Rudolf Steiner in 1919; their growth in the past ten years has been phenomenal. There is probably a Waldorf preschool near you.[8] If so, we encourage you to visit it and see for yourself. Otherwise you can write to Informed Birth and Parenting for further information.

Stayin' Alive

The best thing that parents can do for young children is to provide a model worthy of imitation. This means watching your temper and your language and your gestures around the young child. It means creating an aura of peace and harmony as best you can. It means working on yourself to the extent that you want to influence the child.

Inner work and transformation have been central to this book. This can involve emotional house-cleaning and achieving as much clarity as possible in relation to your past and your present relationships. It can also mean giving credence to your spiritual longings and setting aside time in a busy schedule for weekly or daily religious services or spiritual practices. Meditation, inner calm, a walk in the woods, can all be very helpful on the path of parenting. The arts can also give energy. A mother who is exhausted from trying to take care of a two-year-old will find that painting, working in clay or playing a musical instrument can actually give her energy—the kind of energy that her child is constantly taking from her.

In serious spiritual work on oneself, there is the "way of the monk" in which a man or woman renounces the world and joins a cloister or monastery to realize union with God. But there is also the "way of the householder" for those who have chosen to do inner work while staying in the world. For those of us who are in the world, let us undertake to continue our own inner growth past the growth and gradual decline of the physical body. In this task our children are our teachers, affording us numerous glimpses into the spiritual world and into our own shortcomings. Let us endeavor to study and understand the human being, so we can both fulfill our own destinies and help our children on the path to fulfilling theirs, knowing that they are not "ours" and that we are only able to help them for a short time. The path is not easy, but the growth is worthwhile!

Appendix

Resource Groups

American Academy of Husband-Coached Childbirth
Box 5224
Sherman Oaks, CA 91413
Provides information on training in the Bradley
method of childbirth for parents and teachers.

American Society for Psychoprophylaxis in
   Obstetrics (ASPO)
1411 K Street N.W.
Washington, DC 20005
Provides information on training in the Lamaze
method of childbirth for parents and teachers.

Association for Childbirth at Home International
P.O. Box 39498
Los Angeles, CA 90039
Provides information on home birth for parents and
teachers.

Cesarean Prevention Movement
P.O. Box 152, University Station
Syracuse, NY 13210
Information on preventing unnecessary cesareans.

C/Sec
22 Forest Road
Framingham, MA 01701
Support for those who have had a Cesarean section,
or those who want to avoid one.

Couple to Couple League
P.O. Box 11084
Cincinnati, OH 45211
Information and training in natural birth control.

The Farm
156 Drake's Lane
Summertown, TN 39483
Books and quarterly journal, *The Birth Gazette.*

Informed Homebirth/Informed Birth and Parenting
P.O. Box 3675
Ann Arbor, MI 48106
Information on training in birth alternatives for
parents and teachers; newsletter; childbirth educator
certification and midwifery skills workshops.

International Childbirth Education Association
   (ICEA)
P.O. Box 20048
Minneapolis, MN 55420
Information on preparation for family-centered
maternity care for parents and teachers.

La Leche League International
9616 Minneapolis Avenue
Franklin Park, IL 60131
Information and support for breastfeeding—check
for local chapters.

March of Dimes
Information and support on birth defects—check for
local chapters.

Midwives Alliance of North America
P.O. Box 1121
Bristol, VA 24203
Information on midwifery, newsletter, conferences.

Mothers of Twins Club
5402 Amberwood Lane
Rockville, MD 20853
Newsletter and support.

National Association of Parents and Professionals for
   Safe Alternatives in Childbirth (NAPSAC)
P.O. Box 429
Marble Hill, MO 63764
Directory of Alternative Birth Services, books,
newsletter.

Parent to Parent
NICU Follow Up Clinic
San Francisco Children's Hospital
3700 California Street
San Francisco, CA 94118
Support for parents of premature and other neonatal intensive care unit (NICU) babies—check your hospital for similar support groups.

Further Reading

Pregnancy and Childbirth

A Child is Born, Lennart Nilsson
Magnificent photos of fetal development—a must to see.

Birth Without Violence, Frederick LeBoyer
LeBoyer's insights into the need for gentle childbirth; well illustrated and written.

Childbirth with Insight, Elizabeth Noble
This book encourages women to leave behind "methods" and let go to give birth naturally.

Childbirth Without Fear, Grantly Dick-Read, M.D.
A classic in childbirth education theory by a pioneer in the movement for prepared natural childbirth.

The Complete Book of Pregnancy and Childbirth,
   Sheila Kitzinger
A comprehensive book by a well-known leader in childbirth education.

The Dream Worlds of Pregnancy, Eileen Stukane
Increases awareness and insight into pregnant mothers' and fathers' dreams.

Giving Birth: Parents' Emotions During Labor and Childbirth, Sheila Kitzinger
Cases of clinic/hospital births from Great Britain.

A Good Birth, A Safe Birth, Diana Korte and
   Roberta Scaer
A woman-oriented guide to creating the birth you want.

Husband-Coached Childbirth, Robert Bradley, M.D.
Helpful background on the Bradley method of childbirth—if you can get past his patronizing attitude towards women.

Right from the Start, Gail Brewer and Janice Greene
Excellent guide to present-day childbirth, especially for those choosing hospital or birth center births.

Safe Alternatives in Childbirth, Five Standards of Safe Childbearing, Twentieth-Century Obstetrics Now, NAPSAC
Some excellent publications available from an active national organization.

Special Delivery, Rahima Baldwin
Clear and comprehensive guide for natural/home birth. Required reading for all birthing couples.

Spiritual Midwifery, Ina May Gaskin
An inspiring home birth book, written by a midwife in a large, alternative community where natural home birth is the norm. Many birth stories included.

Transformation Through Birth, Claudia Panuthos
This is an excellent book about being aware and growing during pregnancy.

The Whole Birth Catalog, Janet Isaacs Ashford, ed.
A sourcebook for choices in childbirth.

Special Concerns

Children at Birth, Marjie and Jay Hathaway
Warm book about the joy of having siblings at birth and pointers on preparing them for the experience. Home-birth oriented.

Ended Beginnings, Claudia Panuthos and
   Catherine Romeo
A compassionate look at healing loss from abortion, stillbirth, miscarriage, or upsetting birth experiences. The best of its kind.

Essential Exercises for the Childbearing Year,
   Elizabeth Noble
Includes a section on post-cesarean exercises. This book explains why it's important to exercise and how best to do it, by someone who knows. Heartily recommended.

Having Twins, Elizabeth Noble
"How to's" for parenting twins, including how to have full-term, normal-sized ones!

Making Love During Pregnancy, Elizabeth Bing and
    Libby Coleman
Reassurances about changes in sexual desire during
pregnancy and advice for dealing with the changes.

Maternal-Infant Bonding, Marshall Klaus and John
    Kennel
Explains the studies done on bonding and their
significance.

To Love and Let Go, Suzanne Arms
Special help for mothers who will give or have
given a child up for adoption.

The Pregnancy After 30 Workbook, Gail Brewer
Practical guide to questions of women over 30 who
wonder how their age might affect their pregnancy
and birthing. Includes a lot of general information,
helpful to anyone.

A New Look at Birthing

Birth Reborn, Michel Odent, M.D.
This French obstetrician discusses birth in general
and at his clinic in Pithiviers. He presents a model
that really gives birth back to women. Should be
read by all.

Immaculate Deception, Suzanne Arms
Powerful expose of technological birthing in
America.

In Labor: Women & Power in the Birthplace,
    Barbara Katz Rothman
Analyzes current obstetrical practice as compared to
midwifery practices, and how sexism affects it all.

Lying In: A History of Childbirth in America,
    Dorothy and Richard Wertz
The history of male usurpation of the birth process.

*Reclaiming Birth: History and Heroines of
    American Childbirth Reform,* Margot Edwards
    and Mary Waldorf
Traces developments from 1930 to the present,
featuring biographies of seven prominent women.

*Silent Knife: Cesarean Prevention and Vaginal
    Birth After Cesarean,* Nancy Wainer Cohen and
    Lois J. Estner
This is a much-needed book for all of us in a high-
tech society where pregnancy and birth are often
treated as disease by the medical profession.

Videos and Tapes

The following are available from Informed Birth
and Parenting, P.O. Box 3675, Ann Arbor, MI 48106.

Special Delivery, Rahima Baldwin (video)
Shows home, hospital, and birth center births, and
couples discussing their decisions. $39.95.

Five Women/Five Births, Suzanne Arms (video)
Emphasizes women making their own best choices.
Births are in various settings; cesarean and vaginal
breeches included. $49.95.

Birth: A Family Experience, Oracle Video (video)
Homebirth with sibling and grandmother present.
$29.95.

Informed Homebirth Tape Series, Rahima Baldwin
Six cassettes on preparation for homebirth, $40.00.
With the book *Special Delivery* and a year's
membership in Informed Homebirth, $49.75.

Also available:

Reclaiming Midwifery, Michigan Midwives
Association (video)
This video illustrates midwifery care and
homebirth. $30. Order from: Michigan Midwives
Association, Route 1, Hesperia, MI 49421.

Breastfeeding

Breastfeeding Your Baby, Sheila Kitzinger
This comprehensive book is well illustrated with
color photos.

Bestfeeding: Getting Breastfeeding Right for You,
    Mary Renfrew, Chloe Fisher, Suzanne Arms.
This is a book for every new mother to keep by
her side.

The Womanly Art of Breastfeeding, La Leche
    League
A revised edition of the long-time, helpful guide
and encourager of breastfeeding.

*You Can Breastfeed Your Baby, Even in Special
    Situations,* Dorothy Patricia Brewster
Covers special situations such as twins, premature
babies, working mothers, and many more.

Nutrition

Diet for a Small Planet, Frances Lappe
Good nutrition without eating animals—an economical, conscious and healthy choice—is given with many delicious recipes and information on food combining to make complete proteins.

Vegetarian Baby, Sharon Intema
For those with a vegetarian lifestyle, here is evidence, support, and advice on how to raise a healthy vegetarian child, beginning with pregnancy.

What Every Pregnant Woman Should Know,
   Gail Sforza Brewer
This book explains toxemia, and why diuretics and avoiding salt can cause problems during pregnancy, even though they are often prescribed to "prevent" toxemia. Explains nutritional guidelines for preventing toxemia.

Childcare and Mothering

Growing Up Free: Raising Your Child in the 80's,
   Letty Cottin Pogrebin
Practical and theoretical guide to raising free, nonsexist children. It also explains why nonsexist child-rearing is better for everyone.

Healing At Home, A Guide to Health Care for
   Children, Mary Howell, M.D.
Excellent book for those who want to take some responsibility for the health care of their family.

Momma: A Source book for Single Mothers, edited
   by Karol Hope and Nancy Young
Advice for those who are single on forming support systems, as well as other practical ideas.

The Mother's Book, edited by Ronnie Friedland and
   Carol Kort
This book includes the stories of many different pregnancies, births, and mothering experiences as told by the mothers themselves. It includes the dark side, as well as the light.

Mothering Magazine, Box 8410, Santa Fe, NM
   87504
Excellent quarterly magazine, especially for those who aspire to live a natural lifestyle.

Mothercare, Lyn Deliquadri and Kathi Breckenridge
A must for all pregnant women to read—how to take care of *yourself,* as well as the family, post-partum.

Of Woman Born: Motherhood as Experience and
   Institution, Adrienne Rich
A feminist view of motherhood which includes awareness of its essence, as well as its imposed stereotypes.

Ourselves and Our Children, Boston Women's
   Health Book Collective
Insightful book for helping us see ourselves in relation to our children.

The Well Baby Book and *The Well Child Book,*
   Mike Samuels, M.D. and Nancy Samuels
Basic books to consult in deciding when to get more expert help and when to treat at home. Holistic health care at its best. *The Well Child Book* includes educational section on anatomy and physiology written for children.

Whole Child/Whole Parent, Polly Berends
A spiritual guide to the learning process of being a parent and raising a child. Includes many practical hints, toys, and book reviews.

You Are Your Child's First Teacher, Rahima Baldwin
Parenting and child development from birth through age six. Draws from the insights of Rudolf Steiner.

Special Concerns of Childcare

"Circumcision Packet" and "Immunization Packet,"
   Mothering Magazine.
These two information packets include articles which have appeared over several years in *Mothering,* both pro and con. Helpful in making informed decisions.

Circumcision: The Painful Dilemma,
   Rosemary Romberg
A comprehensive study of all aspects of the issue.

Infant Massage, Vimala Schneider
A leader in infant massage, Vimala adapts techniques from India. Well illustrated.

Loving Hands, Frederick LeBoyer
Inspiring photos of traditional infant massage in India.

The Magical Child, Joseph Chilton Pearce
A beautiful book that challenges childrearing theories with a new way of looking at learning.

Waldorf (Steiner) Education and Related Books

Better Late than Early, Raymond and
      Dorothy Moore
Arguments supporting the delay of cognitive school
work.

Conception, Birth and Early Childhood,
    Norbert Glas
Includes spiritual and practical considerations to
develop understanding of the nature of the child
and its need for protection of the senses.

*Early Childhood Education and the Waldorf School
    Plan,* Elizabeth Grunelius
Description of the nature of early childhood and a
typical Waldorf preschool by the first Waldorf kindergarten teacher.

The Education of the Child, Rudolf Steiner
Describes the physical and less tangible
development of the child and how education needs
to be different for different ages.

Festivals, Family and Food, Diana Carey and
    Judy Large
Suggestions for enhancing family life through the
festivals of the year.

The Four Temperaments, Rudolf Steiner
Description of the sanguine, melancholic, choleric
and phlegmatic temperaments and how a teacher
might work differently with each.

The Hurried Child, David Elkind
This psychologist shows the damage caused by the
pressure to grow up too soon exerted by schools,
parents, the media and our whole society today.

The Kingdom of Childhood, Rudolf Steiner
Steiner details the different seven-year cycles of
development and how the child should be met at
each age.

The Recovery of Man in Childhood, A. C. Harwood
Excellent introduction to Steiner's view of the
human being and principles of education.

Waldorf Parenting Handbook, Lois Cusick
Easily understandable guide to the development of
the child and the way the Waldorf schools teach the
various ages.

The Way of a Child, A. C. Harwood
An excellent first book for those interested in the
Waldorf view of the child and child development.

You Are Your Child's First Teacher, Rahima Baldwin
See preceding page.

Woman-Care

Breasts, Daphna Ayalah and Isaac Weinstock
Women discuss their breasts and their lives—
amazing book.

Wisewoman Herbal for the Childbearing Year,
Susun Weed
Recommendations for pregnancy, birth and
postpartum by an experienced herbalist.

Hygieia, A Woman's Herbal, Jeannine Parvati
The use of herbs and the nature of healing throughout a woman's life.

How to Stay out of the Gynecologist's Office, The
    Federation of Feminist Women's Health Centers
Excellent practical guide to women's health and self-
help.

A New View of a Woman's Body, The Federation of
    Feminist Women's Health Centers
Richly illustrated guide covering self-examination,
birth control, health problems, and more.

Mal(e) Practice (How Doctors Manipulate Women),
    Robert S. Mendelsohn, M.D.
How to avoid being patronized by doctors, written
by the "Medical Heretic."

The New Our Bodies, Our Selves, The Boston
    Women's Health Book Collective
Newly revised and expanded, on all aspects of
women's health, relationships, fertility, and more.

Women's Experience of Sex, Sheila Kitzinger
This noted author records women's experiences in
all phases of their life cycle. Very powerful book.

Footnotes

Chapter 1   Trusting Birth

1. Ina May Gaskin, *Spiritual Midwifery* (Summertown, TN: The Book Publishing Company, 1978).
2. Elizabeth Davis, *Heart and Hands: A Midwife's Guide,* (Berkeley, CA: Celestial Arts, 1987, p. 2).
3. Zelda Stern, "The Healing Touch," *Childbirth Educator,* Vol. 4, No. 4, Summer 1985, p. 45.
4. Dolores Krieger, *The Therapeutic Touch: How to Use Your Hands to Help or Heal* (Englewood Cliffs, NJ: Prentice-Hall, 1979).
5. Stern, *op.cit.,* p 47.
6. Niles Newton, "Childbirth and Culture," *Psychology Today,* November 1970, p. 75.
7. Dr. Michel Odent, *Birth Reborn* (New York, NY: Pantheon Books, 1984, p. 45).
8. A point first made by Cybele Gold in *Joyous Childbirth. A Manual for Conscious Natural Childbirth* (Berkeley, CA: And/Or Press, 1977).
9. Kathleen Stocking. "The Rebirth of Home Birth," *MICHIGAN. The Magazine of the Detroit News,* February 12, 1984, p. 13.
10. *Ibid,* p. 14.
11. Thomas Verny, M.D. with John Kelly, *The Secret Life of the Unborn Child* (New York, NY: Summit Books, 1981).
12. Nancy Wainer Cohen and Lois Estner, *Silent Knife. Cesarean Prevention and Vaginal Birth after Cesarean.,* (South Hadley, MA: Bergin & Garvey, 1983, p. 41).
13. Dr. O. Carl Simonton, Stephanie Matthews-Simonton, and James Creighton, *Getting Well Again* (New York, NY: Bantam Books, 1980).
14. Gayle Peterson with contributions by Lewis Mehl, M.D., *Birthing Normally: A Personal Growth Approach to Childbirth* (Berkeley, CA: Mind/Body Press, 1981).
15. Grantley Dick-Read, *Childbirth Without Fear,* rev., 4th ed. (New York, NY: Harper Row, 1978).
16. Peterson, *op. cit.*

Chapter 2   Changing Feelings/Feeling Changes

1. Eileen Stukane, *The Dream Worlds of Pregnancy* (New York, NY: Quill, 1985).
2. *Ibid,* p. 121.
3. Judith Lamley, Ph.D., "The Image of the Fetus in the First Trimester," *Birth and the Family Journal,* Vol. 7:1, Spring 1980, pp. 5-14.
4. Verny, *op. cit.*
5. Lennart Nilsson et al, *A Child is Born: The Drama of Life Before Birth* (New York, NY: Dell Publishing, 1969).
6. Daphna Ayalah and Isaac Weinstock, *Breasts.* (New York, NY: Summit Books, 1979).
7. Gail Brewer with Tom Brewer, M.D., *What Every Pregnant Woman Should Know: The Truth about Diet and Drugs in Pregnancy* (New York, NY: Random House, rev. 1985).
8. Marilyn Moran, *Birth and the Dialogue of Love* (Leewood, KS: New Nativity Press, 1981).
9. Elizabeth Bing and Libby Colman, *Making Love During Pregnancy* (New York, NY: Bantam, 1977).
10. Nancy Friday, *My Mother/My Self* (NY: Dell, 1977).
11. Phoenix Institute, *The Assertive Workbook: A Guide to Assertive Behavior* (Salt Lake City, UT: Phoenix Institute, 1978, p. 202).
12. Claudia Panuthos, *Transformation through Birth* (South Hadley, MA: Bergin & Garvey, 1984).
13. Colette Dowling, *The Cinderella Complex: Women's Hidden Fear of Independence* (New York, NY: Summit Books, 1981).

Chapter 3   Birth: Images and Reality

1. Cohen and Estner, *op. cit.*
2. Panuthos, *op. cit.*
3. Cohen and Estner, *op. cit.,* p. 120.
4. Richard and Dorothy Wertz, *Lying-In: A History of Childbirth in America* (New York, NY: Macmillan, 1977).
5. 1987 World Population Data Sheet. *Mothering Magazine,* Summer 1988, p. 63.
6. Robert Bradley, M.D., *Husband-Coached Childbirth* (New York, NY: Harper & Row, 1974).
7. Fernand Lamaze, M.D., *Painless Childbirth: The Lamaze Method* (New York, NY: Pocket Books, 1972).
8. Sheila Kitzinger, *The Experience of Childbirth,* 5th ed. (New York, NY: Penguin, 1984).
9. Gayle Peterson, *op. cit.*
10. Rahima Baldwin, *Special Delivery* (Berkeley, CA: Celestial Arts, 1979).
11. Ina May Gaskin, *Spiritual Midwifery* (Summertown, TN: The Book Publishing Company, 1978).
12. R. Sosa, J. Kennell, M. Klaus, S. Robertson, and J. Urrutia, "The Effect of a Supportive Companion on Perinatal Problems, Length of Labor, and Mother-Infant Interaction." *New England Journal of Medicine,* 303:597-600, 1980.

13. Sheila Kitzinger, unpublished address at the ICEA International Convention, St. Louis, MO, June 1984.
14. Cohen and Estner, *op. cit.*
15. Carl Haub, *op. cit.*

Chapter 4 Birthing Renaissance

1. Margot Edwards and Mary Waldorf, *Reclaiming Birth: History and Heroines of American Childbirth Reform* (Trumansburg, NY: The Crossing Press, 1984).
2. Odent, *op. cit.*
3. *Ibid,* p. 94.
4. *Birth Reborn,* available in 16mm and video format, for sale or rent from The Texture Films Collection, P.O. Box 1337, Skokie, IL 60076.
5. Odent, *op. cit.,* p. 44.
6. *Ibid,* p. 118.
7. *Ibid,* p. 116.
8. Perinatal mortality is defined here as deaths between 28 weeks gestation and 28 days after birth. See next two footnotes for statistics.
9. Gaskin, *op. cit.,* Appendix.
10. Odent, *op. cit.,* p. 117.
11. *Ibid,* p. 118.
12. Sheila Kitzinger, "Introduction" to Odent, *op. cit.,* p. xix.
13. Adrienne Rich, *Of Woman Born: Motherhood as Experience and Institution,* (Guilford, CT: Norton, 1976, p. 285).

Chapter 5 Recognizing Your Roots

1. Carl Franz, *The People's Guide to Mexico* (Santa Fe, NM: John Muir Press, 1979).
2. Gayle Peterson, *op. cit.*
3. Sheila Kitzinger, *Woman's Experience of Sex* (New York, NY: G.P. Putman's Sons, 1983), p. 132.
4. Panuthos, *op. cit.,* pp. 16–17.
5. Kitzinger, *op. cit.*

Chapter 6 Becoming a Clear Channel for Birth

1. Elizabeth Depperman Gilmore, "Facing the Worst," *Mothering,* No. 16, Spring, 1980.
2. Carl Simonton, *op. cit.*
3. Claudia Panuthos and Catherine Romeo, *Ended Beginnings* (South Hadley, MA: Bergin & Garvey, 1985).
4. Peterson, *op. cit.*
5. Leonard Orr and Sondra Ray, *Rebirthing in the New Age* (Berkeley, CA: Celestial Arts, 1978).

6. Elisabeth Kübler-Ross, M.D., *On Death and Dying* (New York, NY: Macmillan, 1969).
7. Panuthos and Romeo, *op. cit.*
8. Kübler-Ross, *op. cit.*
9. Suzanne Arms, *To Love and Let Go* (New York, NY: Alfred Knopf, 1983).
10. Marshall Klaus and John Kennell, *Parent-Infant Bonding* (St. Louis, MO: C.V. Mosby, 1982).
11. Ron Taylor and Jude Bea-Taylor, *Jonah Has a Rainbow. A Film on Premature Birth* (Boulder, CO: Centre Productions, Inc., 1983).
12. Panuthos, *op. cit.,* p. 56.
13. Suzanne Arms, *Immaculate Deception* (New York, NY: Bantam Books, 1975).
14. Cohen and Estner, *op. cit.*
15. *Ibid.*
16. Panuthos, *op. cit.*
17. Peterson, *op. cit.*

Chapter 7 Fulfilling Relationships

1. Leni Schwartz, Ph.D., "The Child Within," six meditations on cassette for $9.95 from 1275 Canyon Rd., Santa Fe, NM 87501.
2. Laura Hersey, "Birthing Tools," 4 cassettes for $29.95 from P.O. Box 1542, Vienna, VA 22180.
3. Gail Brewer, *op. cit.*
4. Information can be researched in the March, 1982 *Lancet,* and September, 1982 *Prevention.* We understand that a drug company is starting to market it in conjunction with other ingredients for morning sickness—watch for it.
5. Shelia Kitzinger, *op. cit.*
6. Jolan Chang, *The Tao of the Loving Couple* (New York, NY: E.P. Dutton, 1983) and *The Tao of Love and Sex* (Dutton, 1977).

Chapter 8 Looking Toward Giving Birth

1. The Informed Homebirth Tape Series includes *Special Delivery* and a year's membership in Informed Homebirth for $49.75. Childbirth educator training is also available through workshops or a Correspondence Program. IH/IBP, Box 3675, Ann Arbor, MI 48106.
2. Elizabeth Noble, *Childbirth with Insight* (Boston, MA: Houghton Mifflin Co., 1983).
3. *The American Heritage Dictionary of the English Language* (Boston, MA: Houghton Mifflin Co., 1979).
4. For a detailed explanation of visualizations and how they work, see Peterson, *op. cit.,* Ch IV.
5. Sheila Kitzinger and Penny Simkin, Eds., *Episiotomy and the Second Stage of Labor* (Seattle, WA: Pennypress, 1984).

6. *Standards of Obstetric-Gynecologic Services* of the American College of Obstetricians and Gynecologists, pp. 66–67.
7. Available from ICEA, P.O. Box 20048, Minneapolis, MN 55420.
8. Janet Isaacs Ashford, ed., *The Whole Birth Catalog* (Trumansburg, NY: The Crossing Press, 1983), pp. 84–88.
9. Cohen and Estner, *op. cit.,* Chs. 13 and 14.
10. Michel Odent, M.D. in a talk, "The Art of Birthing" at Michigan State University, East Lansing, MI, Oct. 29, 1984.
11. Cohen and Estner, *op. cit.,* Ch. 11.
12. Frederick LeBoyer, *Birth Without Violence* (New York, NY: Alfred A. Knopf, 1975.)
13. Studies quoted in Baldwin, *op. cit.,* pp. 6–7.

Chapter 9   Opening to Birth

1. Gaskin, *op. cit.*
2. *Ibid.*
3. Noble, *op. cit.,* p. 73.
4. See studies by Constance Beynon, quoted in Baldwin, *op. cit.,* pp. 88–89.
5. *Birth in the Squatting Position* produced by CPP Pesquises is available from Polymorph Films, 118 South St., Boston, MA 02111.
6. *Ibid.*
7. M. F. Schutte, et. al, "Management of Premature Rupture of Membranes: The Risk of Vaginal Examination to the Infant," *American Journal of Obstetrics and Gynecology,* June 15, 1983, pp. 395–399.
8. Emanual A. Friedman, "Use of Labor Pattern as a Management Guide," Hospital Topics, 46 (No. 8); 58, 1968.
9. Barbara Katz Rothman, *In Labor: Women and Power in the Birth Place* (New York, NY: Norton, 1982).
10. Cohen and Estner, *op. cit.*

Chapter 10   Looking Toward Parenting

1. Robin Morgan, ed., *Sisterhood Is Global* (New York, NY: Doubleday, 1984) pp. 696–99.
2. Gail Sforza Brewer, ed., *The Pregnancy After 30 Workbook* (Emmaus, PA: Rodale Press, 1978).
3. David Elkind, *The Hurried Child* (Reading, MA: Addison-Wesley, 1981).
4. Edward Wallerstein, *Circumcision: An American Health Fallacy* (New York, NY: Springer, 1980).
5. Rosemary Romberg, *Circumcision: The Painful Dilemma* (South Hadley, MA: Bergin & Garvey, 1985).
6. Lyn DelliQuadri and Kathi Breckenridge, *The New Mothercare* (Los Angeles, CA: Jeremy P. Tarcher, Inc., 1984).
7. Marjie and Jay Hathaway, *Children at Birth* (Sherman Oaks, CA: Academy Publications, 1978).
8. Panuthos and Romeo, *op. cit.,* p. 34.

Chapter 11   For New Parents

1. William Wordsworth, "Ode: Intimations of Immortality," from *Recollections of Early Childhood.*
2. Bing and Colman, *op. cit.*
3. Margaret Nofziger, *A Co-operative Method of Natural Birth Control* (Summertown, TN: The Book Publishing Co., 1976).
4. Jeannine Parvati, *Hygieia: A Woman's Herbal* (Monroe, UT: Freestone Press, 1979).
5. Frederick Leboyer, *Birth Without Violence* (New York, NY: Alfred Knopf, 1975)
6. Panuthos and Romeo, *op. cit.*

Chapter 12   For Not-So-New Parents

1. For a detailed description see Rudolf Steiner, *The Four Temperaments* (Spring Valley, NY: Anthroposophic Press, 1968).
2. The recommended pentatonic scale contains no C or F. Children's harps can be ordered from Choroi, 4600 Minnesota Ave., Fair Oaks, CA 95628 or Song of the Sea, 47 West St., Bar Harbor, ME 04609.
3. For further information on how to make such toys, see Freya Jaffke, *Making Soft Toys* (Berkeley, CA: Celestial Arts, 1981).
4. Rudolf Steiner, *The Education of The Child* (London, Rudolf Steiner Press, 1985).
5. David Elkind, *op. cit.*
6. Raymond and Dorothy Moore, *School Can Wait* (Provo, Utah: Brigham Young University Press, 1979) and *Better Late than Early* (New York, NY: Reader's Digest Press, 1975).
7. Rahima Baldwin, "The Magical Years. Some Waldorf Indications for Early Childhood," *Mothering,* No. 32, Summer 1984, pp. 79–83.
8. For a list of schools contact the Waldorf Kindergarten Association of North America, 9500 Brunett Ave., Silver Springs, MD 20901. They also have a bi-annual newsletter.

Index